针灸组合穴全真图解
（中英文对照版）

Illustration of Combination Points
(Chinese – English)

主 编　郭长青　刘乃刚　付伟涛
　　　　郭　妍
副主编　费　飞　任秋兰　胡　波
　　　　张慧方　陶　琳

中国医药科技出版社

图书在版编目（CIP）数据

针灸组合穴治疗常见病全真图解：汉英对照/郭长青等主编．—北京：中国医药科技出版社，2013.5
ISBN 978-7-5067-6045-4

Ⅰ.①针… Ⅱ.①郭… Ⅲ.①针灸疗法-穴位-图解
Ⅳ.①R224.4

中国版本图书馆 CIP 数据核字（2013）第 057792 号

美术编辑 陈君杞
版式设计 郭小平

出版	中国医药科技出版社
地址	北京市海淀区文慧园北路甲 22 号
邮编	100082
电话	发行：010-62227427 邮购：010-62236938
网址	www.cmstp.com
规格	787×1092mm $\frac{1}{32}$
印张	7$\frac{1}{8}$
字数	142 千字
版次	2013 年 5 月第 1 版
印次	2013 年 5 月第 1 次印刷
印刷	三河市腾飞印务有限公司
经销	全国各地新华书店
书号	ISBN 978-7-5067-6045-4
定价	**25.00 元**

本社图书如存在印装质量问题请与本社联系调换

内容提要

《针灸组合穴全真图解》为北京中医药大学针灸推拿学院经验丰富的专家学者,在吸收和借鉴古代文献和现代研究的基础上,结合二十多年的临床经验编写而成。

全书中英对照,共分为七章,分别详细介绍了内科、外科、妇科、男科、儿科、骨伤科、皮肤科、五官科病证的组合穴治疗处方。本书最重要的特点就是图文并茂。我们为每一个组合穴处方均匹配了一张穴位体表图和穴位解剖图,两种穴位图相互比照,便于读者掌握穴位位置及解剖,有助于精准地取穴定位。

本书适宜从事中医针灸临床、教学、科研工作的人员,以及留学生和国外从事针灸相关工作的人员参考使用。

Brief introduction

Ilustration of Combination Point Treatment for Common Diseases is written by the experienced experts and scholars of School of acupuncture and moxibustion, Beijing University of Chinese Medicine. This book is base on the foundation of absorption and reference to the ancient and modern research, and combined with more than 20 years of clinical experience.

The book is Chinese – English bilingual, and was divided into seven chapters, respectively introduces the combination point treatment prescription for internal medicine, surgery, gynecology and Andrology, pediatrics, Tramotology and orthopedics, dermatology, ophthalmology and otorhinolaryngology. Each combination point treatment prescription match two images to locating the points, one for body surface and one for anatomy. Combined use of the two images can help the readers to master the points location and anatomy.

This book is mainly suitable for staff engaged in traditional Chinese medicine, especially in acupuncture and moxibustion.

前言

自从21世纪以来,针灸因其"绿色"、"天然"的特点而越来越被人们所熟知,并成为中国中医药事业走向世界的重要桥梁。

针灸治疗以穴位为根本,各种治疗措施均通过穴位发挥作用,因此,穴位在针灸学中具有非常重要的地位。针灸治病往往不是单个穴位所能解决,而是需要两个或几个穴位。在长期大量的临床实践中,针灸医家不断总结临床经验,认识到某些穴位一起使用可以起到协同作用,提高疗效,从而形成了一些约定俗成的穴组,逐渐形成了组合穴的概念。

组合穴是由相同或相似治疗作用,或协同治疗作用的两个或两个以上穴位组成的穴组,穴组中的穴位相互配合,发挥综合治疗作用。组合穴是历代针灸医家治疗经验的总结,是一笔宝贵的医学财富,整理和挖掘组合穴治疗的宝贵经验,有利于提高针灸的疗效,更好地为广大患者服务。

为了把中医药事业更好地推向国际,我们认真总结二十多年临床经验,编著了这本中英对照的《针灸组合穴治疗常见病全真图解》。本书着重于临床实践,提炼出治疗各科常见疾病的特效组合穴,力求取穴简易而疗效显著。

编者
2013年3月

Preface

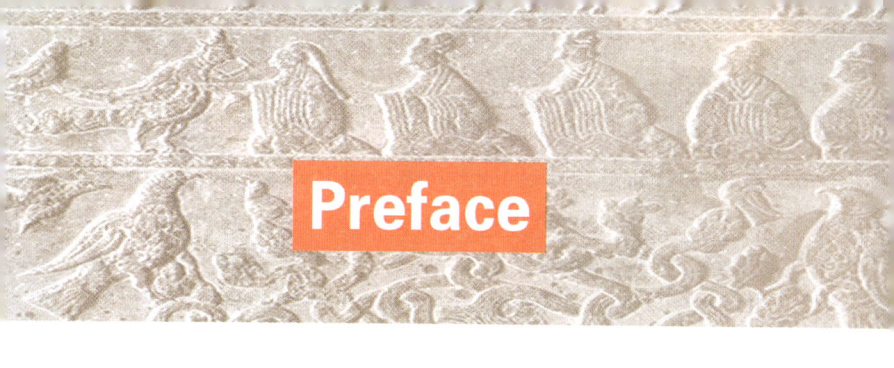

In the 21st century, Acupuncture and moxibustion therapy has got to be known gradually by people all over the world, because of its characteristics of "green", "natural". And become an important bridge for Chinese medicine to the world.

Acupoint is the foundation for Acupuncture and moxibustion therapy, and all treatment play therapeutic roles according to acupoint, therefore, acupoint palys an important role in acupuncture and moxibustion therapy. Freguently, we can not solve problem by a single acupoint, and we need two or more points. In the long – term clinical practice, doctors of acupuncture and moxibustion have accumulated rich experience in clinical practice, they realize that certain acupoints used together have synergy effect and enhance the curative effect, therefore, some specific point groups were established by usage, and the concept of combination point was formed gradually.

combination point is a specific point group formed by two or more acupoints that have similar effects or synergy effect. The acupoints interactions with each other and so as to play a synergistic therapeutic effect. combination points summarized by doctors of acupuncture and moxibustion in the medical clinical practice during a period of long time, and it is a valuable medical wealth. Arranging and mining the valuable experience of combination point is conducive to improve the efficacy of acupuncture and moxibustion, and benefits to serve the patients.

In order to promote the development of traditional Chinese medicine to the world, we summarize the clinical experience for more than 20 years conscientiously, and finally finished the book Ilustration of Combination Point Treatment for Common Diseases (Chinese – English edition). We focuses on clinical practice, and refine some effective combination point for common diseases. we strive to find simple solution and effective in treatment.

March, 2013

目 录

第一章 内科病证
Chapter 1 Medical diseases ……………… 2

第一节 感冒 ……………………………………
Section 1 Common cold   2

第二节 咳嗽 ……………………………………
Section 2 Cough   4

第三节 哮喘 ……………………………………
Section 3 Asthma   6

第四节 胃痛 ……………………………………
Section 4 Gastralgia   8

第五节 胃下垂 …………………………………
Section 5 Gastric ptosis   10

第六节 呕吐 ……………………………………
Section 6 Vomiting   12

第七节 呃逆 ……………………………………
Section 7 Hiccup   14

第八节 腹痛 ……………………………………
Section 8 Bellyache   16

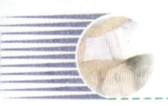

第九节 痢疾 Section 9　Dysentery	18
第十节 便秘 Section 10　Constipation	20
第十一节 胁痛 Section 11　Hypochondria	22
第十二节 黄疸 Section 12　Jaundice	24
第十三节 水肿 Section 13　Edema	26
第十四节 癃闭 Section 14　Retention of urine	28
第十五节 淋证 Section 15　Drench card	30
第十六节 尿失禁 Section 16　Urinary incontinence	32
第十七节 头痛 Section 17　Headache	34
第十八节 三叉神经痛 Section 18　Trigeminal neuralgia	36
第十九节 面瘫 Section 19　Facial paralysis	38
第二十节 面肌痉挛 Section 20　Hemifacial spasm	40
第二十一节 眩晕 Section 21　Vertigo	42

目　录 Directory

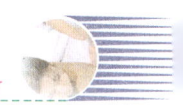

第二十二节　高血压 …………………………… 44
Section 22　Hypertension

第二十三节　低血压 …………………………… 46
Section 23　Hypotension

第二十四节　贫血 ……………………………… 48
Section 24　Anemia

第二十五节　心悸 ……………………………… 50
Section 25　Palpitations

第二十六节　失眠 ……………………………… 52
Section 26　Insomnia

第二十七节　痴呆 ……………………………… 54
Section 27　Dementia

第二十八节　癫病 ……………………………… 56
Section 28　Depressive psychosis

第二十九节　痫病 ……………………………… 58
Section 29　Epilepsy

第三十节　癔病 ………………………………… 60
Section 30　Hysteria

第三十一节　震颤麻痹 ………………………… 62
Section 31　Paralysis agitans

第三十二节　痹证 ……………………………… 64
Section 32　Arthralgia syndrome

第三十三节　腰痛 ……………………………… 78
Section 33　Lumbago

第三十四节　坐骨神经痛 ……………………… 80
Section 34　Sciatica

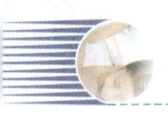

第三十五节 痿证 ………………………………… Section 35　Flaccidity syndrome	82
第三十六节 中风 ………………………………… Section 36　Apoplexy	86
第三十七节 糖尿病 ……………………………… Section 37　Diabetes mellitus	88
第三十八节 单纯性肥胖症 ……………………… Section 38　Simple obesity	90

第二章　外科病证
Chapter 2　Surgical diseases ……………… 92

第一节 疔疮 ……………………………………… Section 1　Malignant furuncle	92
第二节 丹毒 ……………………………………… Section 2　Erysipelas	94
第三节 流行性腮腺炎 …………………………… Section 3　Epidemic parotitis	96
第四节 乳腺炎 …………………………………… Section 4　Mastitis	98
第五节 乳腺增生病 ……………………………… Section 5　Hyperplastic disease of breast	100
第六节 胆石症 …………………………………… Section 6　Cholelithiasis	102
第七节 阑尾炎 …………………………………… Section 7　Appendicitis	104

第八节 疝气 ……………………………… 106
Section 8　Hernia

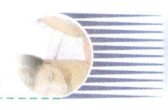

第九节 痔疮 ……………………………… 108
Section 9　Haemorrhoids

第十节 脱肛 ……………………………… 110
Section 10　Prolapse of anus

第三章　妇科、男科病证
Chapter 3　Gynecological and male diseases　……………… 112

第一节 月经不调 ………………………… 112
Section 1　Irregular menstruation

第二节 痛经 ……………………………… 114
Section 2　Dysmenorrhea

第三节 闭经 ……………………………… 116
Section 3　Amenorrhoea

第四节 崩漏 ……………………………… 118
Section 4　Metrorrhagia

第五节 带下病 …………………………… 120
Section 5　Leucorrhoea disease

第六节 阴痒 ……………………………… 122
Section 6　Pruritus vulvae

第七节 子宫脱垂 ………………………… 124
Section 7　Uterine prolapse

第八节 不孕症 …………………………… 126
Section 8　Amenorrhoea

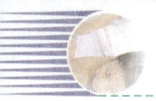

第九节　妊娠呕吐 ………………………………… Section 9　Vomiting of pregnancy	128
第十节　胎位不正 ………………………………… Section 10　Malposition	130
第十一节　滞产 …………………………………… Section 11　Stagnant production	132
第十二节　恶露不绝 ……………………………… Section 12　Prolonged lochia	134
第十三节　产后乳少 ……………………………… Section 13　Postpartum hypogalactia	136
第十四节　围绝经期综合征 ……………………… Section 14　Climacteric syndrome	138
第十五节　经前期紧张综合征 …………………… Section 15　Premenstrual tension syndrome	140
第十六节　遗精 …………………………………… Section 16　Seminal emission	142
第十七节　阳痿 …………………………………… Section 17　Impotence	144
第十八节　早泄 …………………………………… Section 18　Premature ejaculation	146
第十九节　前列腺炎 ……………………………… Section 19　Prostatitis	148
第二十节　男性不育症 …………………………… Section 20　Male infertility	150

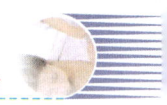

第四章 儿科病证
Chapter 4 Pediatric diseases *152*

第一节 急惊风 ....
Section 1 Acute infantile convulsion
152

第二节 厌食 ....
Section 2 Anorexia
154

第三节 疳证 ....
Section 3 Infantile malnutrition
156

第四节 遗尿 ....
Section 4 Enuresis
158

第五节 多动症 ....
Section 5 Hyperactivity
160

第五章 骨伤科病证
Chapter 5 Orthopedic disorders *162*

第一节 颈椎病 ....
Section 1 Cervical vertebra disease
162

第二节 落枕 ....
Section 2 Have a stiff neck
164

第三节 肩关节周围炎 ....
Section 3 Periarthritis of shoulder
166

第四节 颞下颌关节功能紊乱综合征 ....
Section 4 Temporomandibular joint dysfunction syndrome
168

第五节 肱骨外上髁炎 ....
Section 5 External humeral epicondylitis
170

第六节　跟痛症 …………………………………… *172*
Section 6　Heel pain

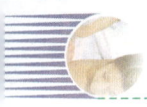

第七节　扭伤 ……………………………………… *174*
Section 7　Sprain

第六章　皮肤科疾病
Chapter 6　Dermatology diseases ………… *186*

第一节　神经性皮炎 ……………………………… *186*
Section 1　Neurodermatitis

第二节　皮肤瘙痒症 ……………………………… *188*
Section 2　Cutaneous pruritus

第三节　荨麻疹 …………………………………… *190*
Section 3　Urticaria

第四节　湿疹 ……………………………………… *192*
Section 4　Eczema

第五节　带状疱疹 ………………………………… *194*
Section 5　Zoster

第六节　痤疮 ……………………………………… *196*
Section 6　Acne

第七节　黄褐斑 …………………………………… *198*
Section 7　Chloasma

第七章　五官科病证
Chapter 7　ENT diseases ………………… *200*

第一节　耳鸣、耳聋 ……………………………… *200*
Section 1　Tinnitus, deafness

第二节　近视 ………………………………… Section 2　Myopia	*202*
第三节　眼睑下垂 ……………………………… Section 3　Ptosis of eyelid	*204*
第四节　眼睑瞤动 ……………………………… Section 4　Eyelid Run dynamic	*206*
第五节　牙痛 …………………………………… Section 5　Toothache	*208*
第六节　咽喉肿痛 ……………………………… Section 6　Sore throat	*210*

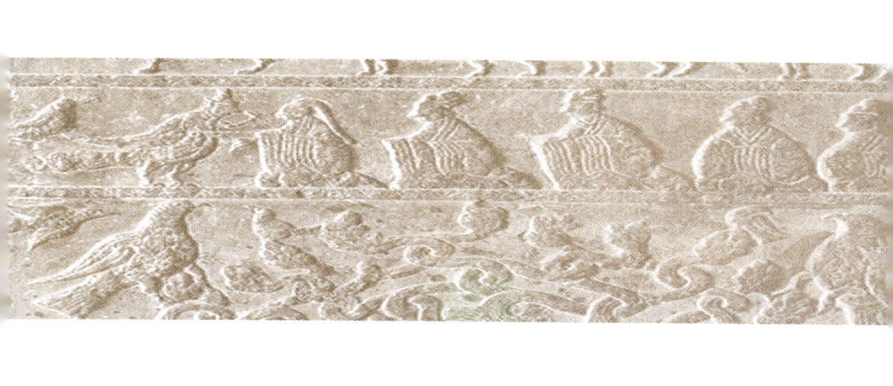

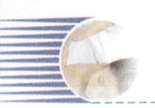

第一章 内科病证
Chapter 1　Medical diseases

第一节　感　冒

组合穴　大椎—风池。

功　能　祛风解表。

大椎

【标准定位】第7颈椎棘突下凹陷中，后正中线上。

【毫针刺法】直刺椎间隙0.8~1.2寸，酸胀或麻电感。

风池

【标准定位】在颈后区，胸锁乳突肌上端与斜方肌上端之间的凹陷中。

【毫针刺法】向鼻尖方向斜刺0.5~1.5寸。

Section 1　Common cold

Combination Point　Dà Zhuī—Fēng Chí.

Actions　Releasing the exterior and expelling wind.

DU 14 Dà Zhuī

Position　On the posterior midline of the neck, in the depression inferior to the spinous process of the seventh cervical vertebra.

Acupuncture　Insert the needle perpendicularly 0.8~1.2 cun deep and stimulate until there is a sore and numbing sensation in the local area.

GB20 Fēng Chí

Position　On the nape, in the depression between m. sternocleidomastoideus and m. trapezius.

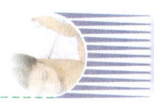

Acupuncture Insert the needle obliquely toward the apex nasi 0.5 ~ 1.5 cun deep.

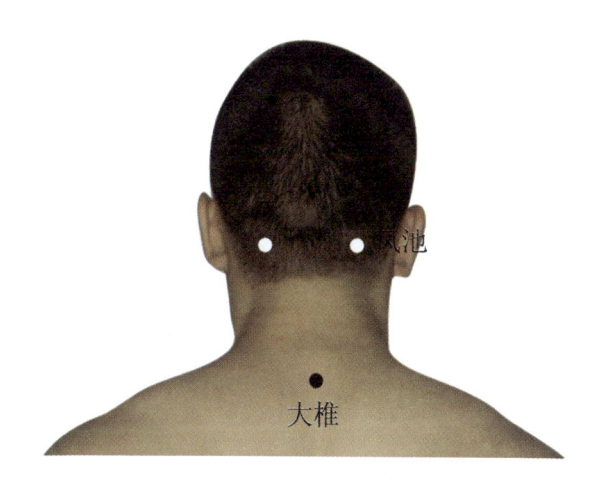

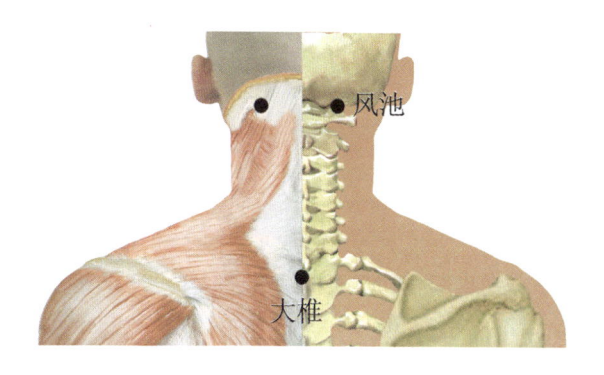

图 1-1 大椎—风池

第二节 咳 嗽

组合穴 列缺—太渊。

功 能 清热疏风,宣肺止咳。

列缺

【标准定位】在前臂,腕掌侧远端横纹上 1.5 寸,拇短伸肌腱与拇长展肌腱之间,拇长展肌肌腱沟的凹陷中。

【毫针刺法】向上斜刺 0.2~0.3 寸,局部酸胀感。

太渊

【标准定位】在腕前区,桡骨茎突与舟状骨之间,拇长展肌腱尺侧凹陷中。

【毫针刺法】直刺 0.2~0.3 寸。

Section 2　Cough

Combination Point　Liè Quē— Tài Yuān.

Actions　Clearing heat and expelling wind, Descending lung qi and alleviating cough.

LU 7 Liè Quē

Position　On the radial side of the forearm, 1.5 cun proximal the transverse crease of the wrist, superior to the styloid process of the radius and between tendons of m. brachioradialis and m. abductor pollicis longus.

Acupuncture　Insert the needle obliquely upward 0.2~0.3 cun deep and stimulate until there is a sore and distending sensation in the local area.

LU 9 Tài Yuān

Position　On the radial end of the wrist crease, where the radial pulse is palpable.

Acupuncture　Insert the needle perpendicularly 0.2~0.3 cun deep.

第一章 内科病证
Chapter 1 Medical diseases

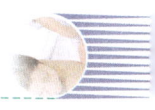

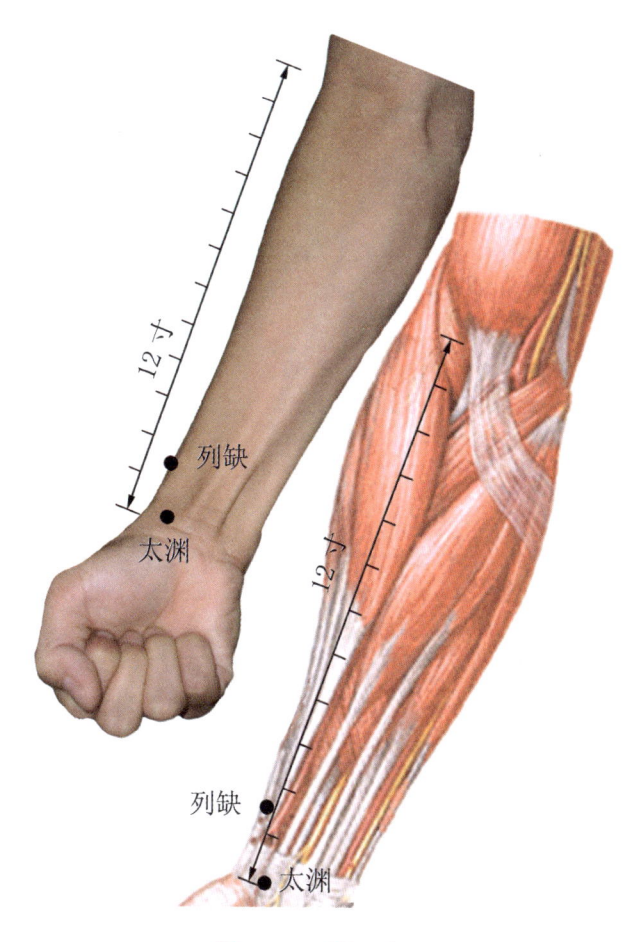

图 1-2 列缺—太渊

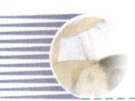

第三节 哮 喘

组合穴 肺俞—定喘。

功 能 宣肺理气,平喘止咳。

肺俞

【标准定位】在背部,第3胸椎棘突下,后正中线旁开1.5寸。

【毫针刺法】向内斜刺0.5~0.8寸,局部酸胀感。

定喘

【标准定位】在脊柱区,第7颈椎棘突下,后正中线旁开0.5寸。

【毫针刺法】直刺或向内斜刺0.5~1寸。

Section 3   Asthma

Combination Point   Fèi Shū— Dìngchuǎn.

Actions   Descending lung qi, alleviating cough and Relieving Asthma.

BL13 Fèi Shū

Position   On the upper back, 1.5 cun lateral to the lower border of the spinous process of the third thoracic vertebra

Acupuncture   Insert the needle obliquely towards the spine 0.5~0.8 cun deep and stimulate until there is a sore and numbing sensation in the local area.

EX – B 5 Dìngchuǎn

Position   On the upper back, 0.5 cun lateral to the lower border of the spinous process of the seventh cervical vertebra.

Acupuncture   Insert the needle perpendicularly or obliquely towards the spine 0.5~1 cun deep.

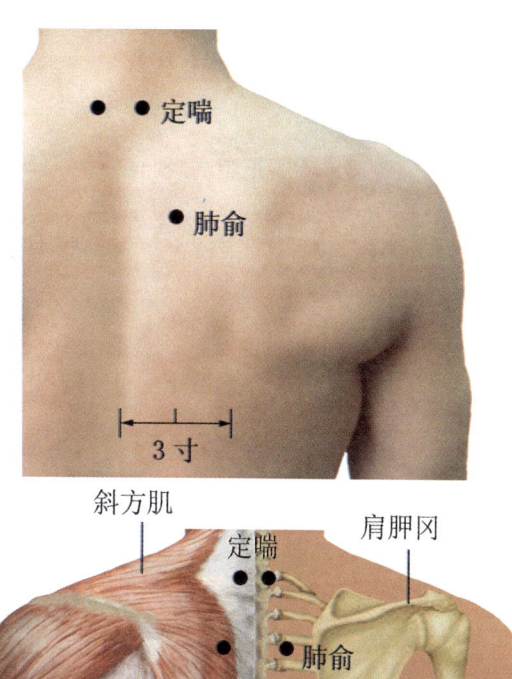

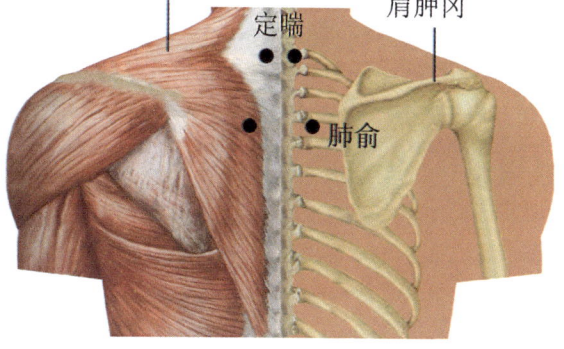

第一章 内科病证
Chapter 1　Medical diseases

定喘

肺俞

3寸

斜方肌　定喘　肩胛冈

肺俞

图1-3　肺俞—定喘

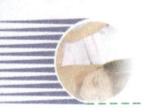

第四节 胃 痛

组合穴 足三里—至阳。

功 能 理气和胃,通络止痛。

足三里

【标准定位】在小腿外侧,犊鼻(ST 35)下3寸,犊鼻(ST 35)与解溪(ST 41)连线上。

【毫针刺法】直刺0.5~1.5寸,局部酸胀。

至阳

【标准定位】在脊柱区,第7胸椎棘突下凹陷中,后正中线上。

【毫针刺法】直刺0.5~1.0寸。

Section 4　Gastralgia

Combination Point　Zú Sān Lǐ— Zhì Yáng.

Actions　Regulating qi and harmonizes the stomach, activating the channel and alleviating pain.

ST36 Zú Sān Lǐ

Position　On the anterior aspect of the lower leg, 3 cun distal to ST 35 (dú bí), one finger width lateral from the anterior ridge of the tibia.

Acupuncture　Insert the needle perpendicularly 0.5 ~ 1.5 cun deep and stimulate until there is a sore and distending sensation.

DU 9 Zhì Yáng

Position　On the posterior midline of the back, in the depression inferior to the spinous process of the seventh thoracic vertebra.

Acupuncture　Insert the needle perpendicularly or obliquely 0.5 ~ 1.0 cun deep.

第一章　内科病证
Chapter 1　Medical diseases

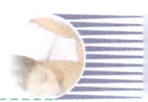

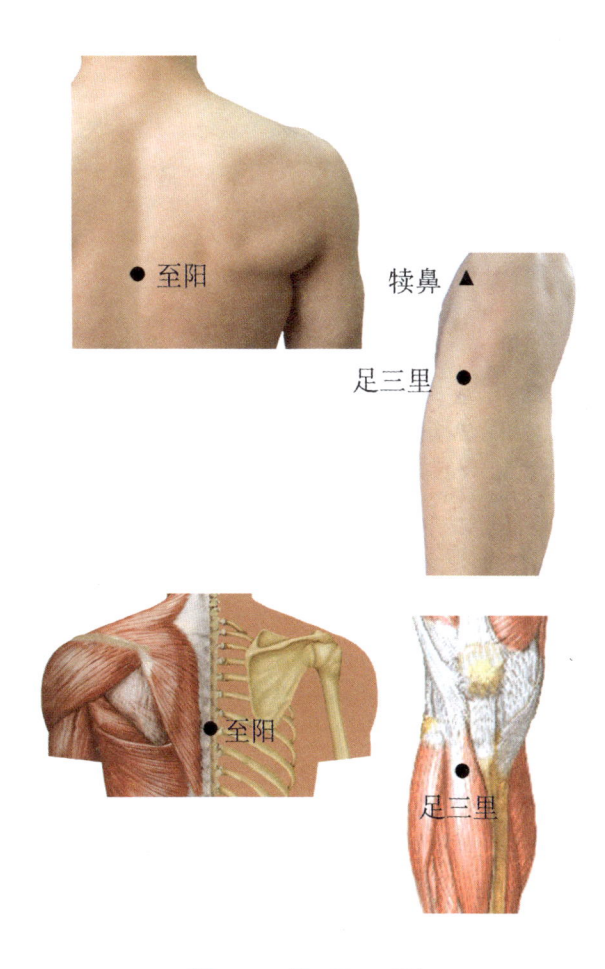

图1-4　足三里—至阳

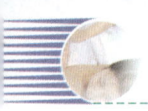

第五节 胃下垂

组合穴 中脘—关元。
功 能 温中补气。

中脘
【标准定位】在上腹部,脐中上4寸,前正中线上。
【毫针刺法】直刺0.5~1.0寸,局部酸胀沉重。

关元
【标准定位】在下腹部,脐中下3寸,前正中线上。
【毫针刺法】需排尿后进行针刺。直刺0.5~1.0寸,局部酸胀,可放射至外生殖器和会阴部。

Section 5 Gastric ptosis

Combination Point Zhōng Wǎn —Guān Yuán.
Actions Warming middle jiao and descending rebellious qi.

RN12 Zhōng Wǎn

Position On the upper abdomen, on the anterior midline, 4 cun superior to the umbilicus.

Acupuncture Insert the needle perpendicularly 0.5~1.0 cun deep and stimulate until there is a sore and distending sensation in the local area.

RN4 Guān Yuán

Position On the lower abdomen, on the anterior midline, 3 cun inferior to the umbilicus.

Acupuncture Insert the needle after the micturition, perpendicularly 0.5~1.0 cun deep and stimulate until there is a sore and distending sensation in the local area radiating to the genitalia.

第一章 内科病证
Chapter 1 Medical diseases

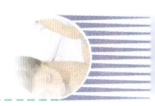

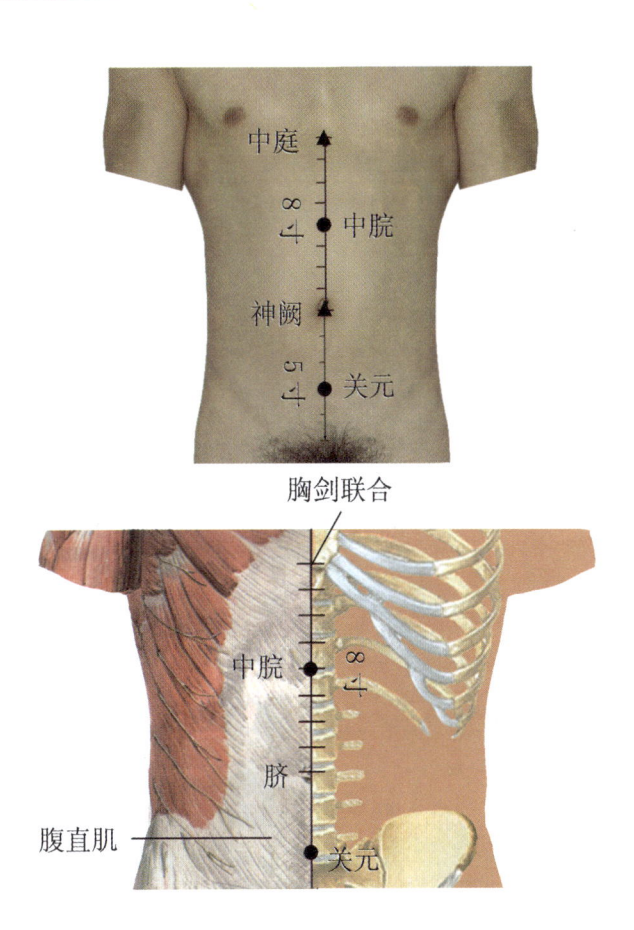

图1-5 中脘—关元

第六节 呕 吐

组合穴 中脘—足三里。

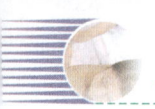

功 能 理气和胃,降逆止呕。

中脘

【标准定位】在上腹部,脐中上4寸,前正中线上。

【毫针刺法】直刺0.5~1.0寸,局部酸胀沉重。

足三里

【标准定位】在小腿外侧,犊鼻(ST 35)下3寸,犊鼻(ST 35)与解溪(ST 41)连线上。

【毫针刺法】直刺0.5~1.5寸,局部酸胀。

Section 6 Vomiting

Combination Point Zhōng Wǎn—Zú Sān Lǐ.

Actions Regulating qi and alleviating vomiting.

RN12 Zhōng Wǎn

Position On the upper abdomen, on the anterior midline, 4 cun superior to the umbilicus.

Acupuncture Insert the needle perpendicularly 0.5 ~ 1.0 cun deep and stimulate until there is a sore and distending sensation in the local area.

ST36 Zú Sān Lǐ

Position On the anterior aspect of the lower leg, 3 cun distal to ST 35 (dú bí), one finger width lateral from the anterior ridge of the tibia.

Acupuncture Insert the needle perpendicularly 0.5 ~ 1.5 cun deep and stimulate until there is a sore and distending sensation.

图 1-6 中脘—足三里

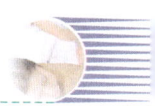

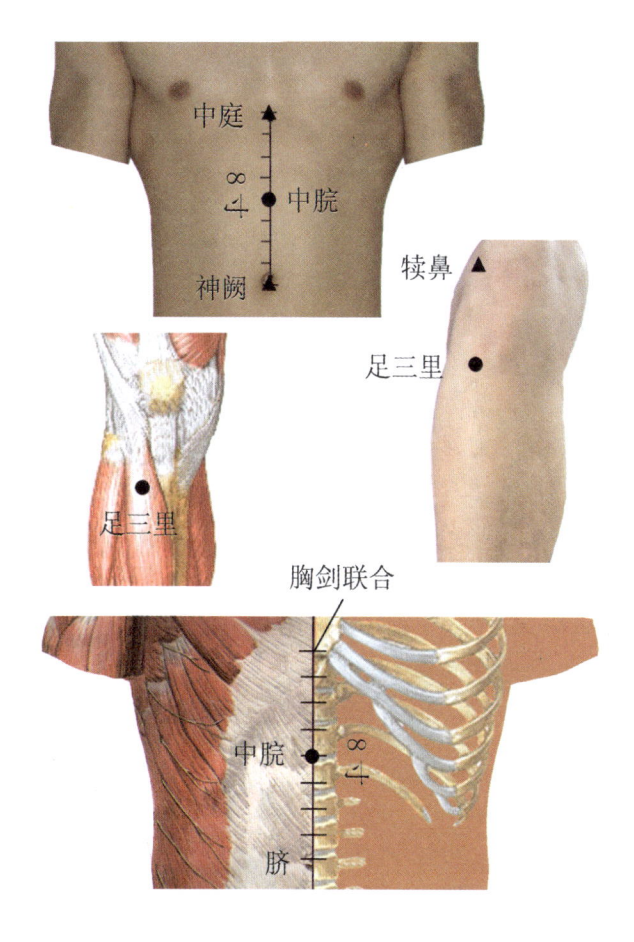

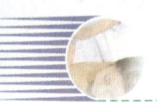

第七节　呃　逆

组合穴　内关—足三里。
功　能　降气止呃。

内关

【标准定位】在前臂前区,腕掌侧远端横纹上2寸,掌长肌腱与桡侧腕屈肌腱之间。

【毫针刺法】直刺0.5~1.5寸,局部酸胀。

足三里

【标准定位】在小腿外侧,犊鼻(ST 35)下3寸,犊鼻(ST 35)与解溪(ST 41)连线上。

【毫针刺法】直刺0.5~1.5寸,局部酸胀。

Section 7　Hiccup

Combination Point　Nèi Guān—Zú Sān Lǐ.

Actions　descending qi and alleviating hiccup.

PC 6 Nèi Guān

Position　On the palmar aspect of the forearm, 2 cun superior to the transverse crease of the wrist, between palmaris longus tendon and flexor carpi radialis tendon.

Acupuncture　Insert the needle perpendicularly 0.5~1.5 cun deep and stimulate until there is a sore and numbing sensation.

ST36 Zú Sān Lǐ

Position　On the anterior aspect of the lower leg, 3 cun distal to ST 35 (dú bí), one finger width lateral from the anterior ridge of the tibia.

Acupuncture　Insert the needle perpendicularly 0.5~1.5 cun deep and stimulate until there is a sore and distending sensation.

图1-7 内关—足三里

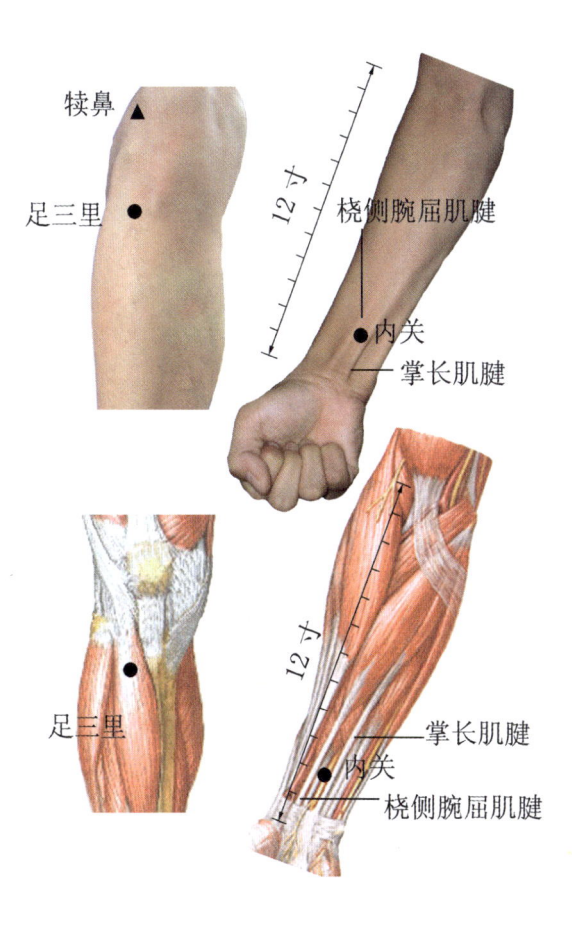

第八节 腹 痛

组合穴 天枢—中脘。

功 能 调中和胃,理气健脾。

天枢

【标准定位】腹部,横平脐中,前正中线旁开2寸。

【毫针刺法】直刺1.0~1.5寸,局部酸胀。

中脘

【标准定位】在上腹部,脐中上4寸,前正中线上。

【毫针刺法】直刺0.5~1.0寸,局部酸胀沉重。

Section 8   Bellyache

Combination Point   Tiān Shū—Zhōng Wǎn.

Actions   Harmonizing stomach and descending rebellious qi.

ST 25 Tiān Shū

Position   On the abdomen, 2 cun lateral to the umbilicus.

Acupuncture   Insert the neelde perpendicularly 1.0 ~ 1.5 cun deep and stimulate until there is a sore and numbing sensation in the local area.

RN12 Zhōng Wǎn

Position   On the upper abdomen, on the anterior midline, 4 cun superior to the umbilicus.

Acupuncture   Insert the needle perpendicularly 0.5 ~ 1.0 cun deep and stimulate until there is a sore and distending sensation in the local area.

图1-8 天枢—中脘

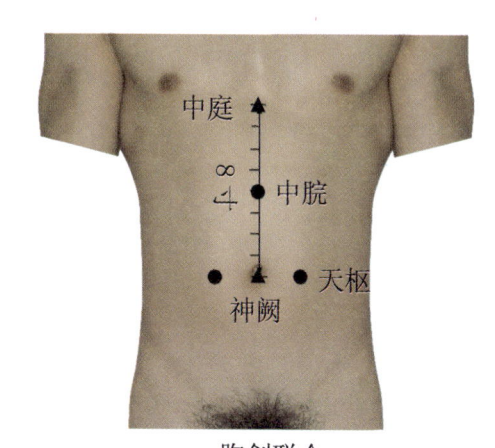

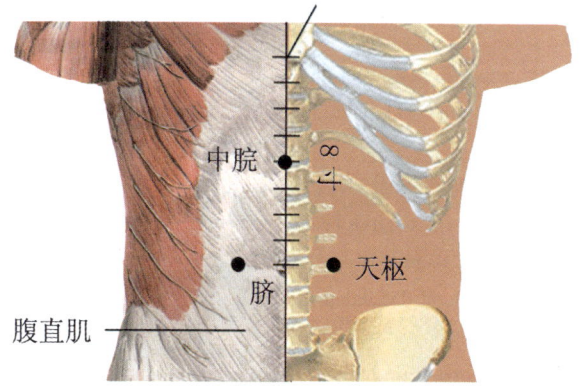

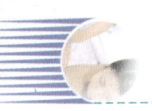

第九节　痢　疾

组合穴　天枢—合谷。

功　能　调肠理气。

天枢

【标准定位】在腹部，横平脐中，前正中线旁开2寸。

【毫针刺法】直刺1.0~1.5寸，局部酸胀，可扩散至同侧腹部。

合谷

【标准定位】在手背，第1、2掌骨间，第2掌骨桡侧的中点处。

【毫针刺法】直刺0.5~1.0寸。

Section 9　Dysentery

Combination Point　Tiān Shū—Hé Gǔ.

Actions　Harmonizing large intestine and regulating qi.

ST 25 Tiān Shū

Position　On the abdomen, 2 cun lateral to the umbilicus.

Acupuncture　Insert the neelde perpendicularly 1.0~1.5 cun deep and stimulate until there is a sore and numbing sensation in the local area radiating to the side of the abdomen.

LI 4 Hé Gǔ

Position　On the dorsum of the hand, between the first and second metacarpal bones, on the radial side of the middle of the second metacarpal bone.

Acupuncture　Insert the needle perpendicularly 0.5~1.0 cun deep.

第一章 内科病证
Chapter 1 Medical diseases

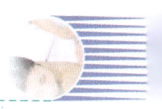

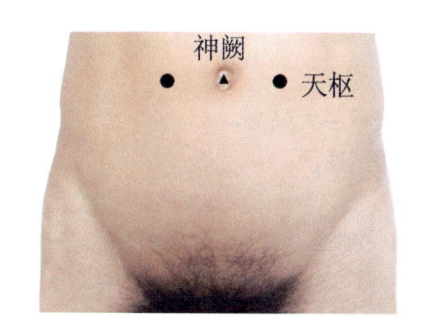

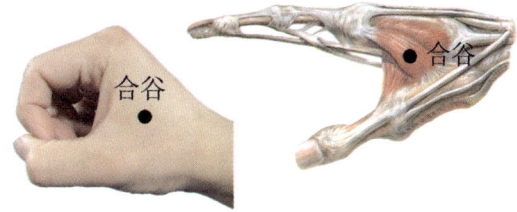

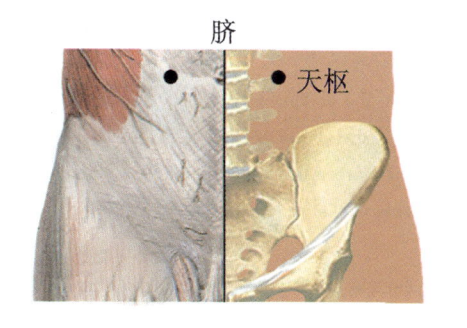

图1-9 天枢—合谷

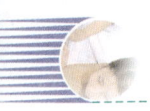

第十节 便 秘

组合穴 天枢—大肠俞。
功 能 理气通便。

天枢
【标准定位】在腹部,横平脐中,前正中线旁开2寸。
【毫针刺法】直刺1.0~1.5寸,局部酸胀,可扩散至同侧腹部。

大肠俞
【标准定位】第4腰椎棘突下,后正中线旁开1.5寸。
【毫针刺法】直刺0.8~1.0寸。

Section 10 Constipation

Combination Point Tiān Shū—Dà Cháng Shū.

Actions Regulating qi and Smoothing Bowels.

ST 25 Tiān Shū

Position On the abdomen, 2 cun lateral to the umbilicus.

Acupuncture Insert the neelde perpendicularly 1.0~1.5 cun deep and stimulate until there is a sore and numbing sensation in the local area radiating to the side of the abdomen.

BL 25 Dà Cháng Shū

Position On the lower back, 1.5 cun lateral to the lower border of the spinous process of the fourth lumbar vertebra.

Acupuncture Insert the needle perpendicularly 0.8~1.0 cun deep.

第一章 内科病证
Chapter 1　Medical diseases

神阙　天枢

腰阳关
大肠俞

脐　天枢

大肠俞

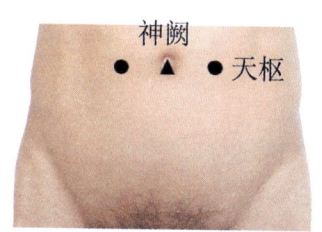

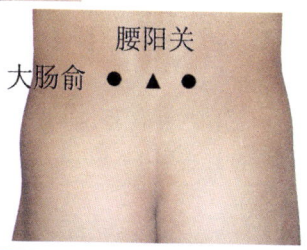

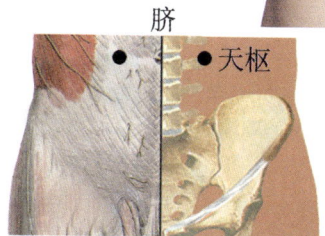

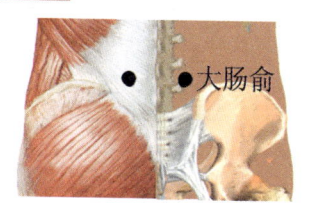

图1-10　天枢—大肠俞

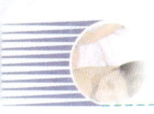

第十一节 胁 痛

组合穴 期门—章门。

功 能 疏肝解郁,理气降逆。

期门
【标准定位】第6肋间隙,前正中线旁开4寸。
【毫针刺法】斜刺0.5~0.8寸,局部酸胀。

章门
【标准定位】在第11肋游离端下方。
【毫针刺法】斜刺0.5~0.8寸。

Section 11   Hypochondria

Combination Point   Qī Mén—Zhāng Mén.

Actions   Spreading liver and regulating qi.

LV14 Qī Mén

Position   On the chest, directly inferior to the nipple, in the sixth intercostal space, 4 cun lateral to the anterior midline.

Acupuncture   Insert the needle obliquely or along the intercostals space 0.5~0.8cun deep and stimulate until there is a sore and numbing sensation in the local area.

LV 13 Zhāng Mén

Position   On the lateral aspect of the abdomen, below the free end of the eleventh floating rib.

Acupuncture   Insert the needle obliquely 0.5~0.8 cun deep.

图 1-11 期门—章门

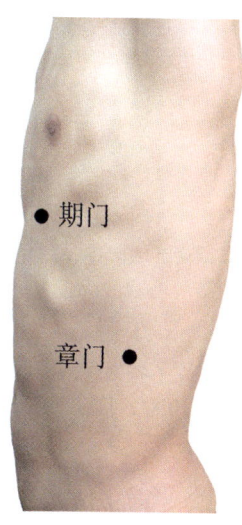

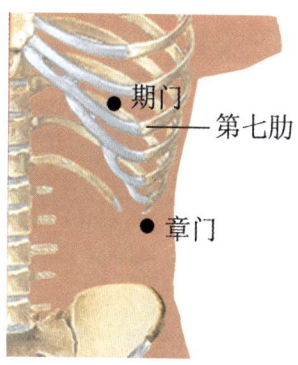

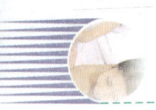

第十二节 黄 疸

组合穴 大椎—至阳。
功 能 清利湿热。

大椎
【标准定位】第 7 颈椎棘突下凹陷中,后正中线上。
【毫针刺法】直刺椎间隙 0.8~1.2 寸,局部酸胀。

至阳
【标准定位】在脊柱区,第 7 胸椎棘突下凹陷中,后正中线上。
【毫针刺法】斜刺 0.5~1.0 寸,局部酸胀。

Section 12　Jaundice

Combination Point　Dà Zhuī— Zhì Yáng.

Actions　Clearing dampness and heat.

DU 14 Dà Zhuī

Position　On the posterior midline of the neck, in the depression inferior to the spinous process of the seventh cervical vertebra.

Acupuncture　Insert the needle perpendicularly 0.8~1.2 cun deep and stimulate until there is a sore and numbing sensation in the local area.

DU 9 Zhì Yáng

Position　On the posterior midline of the back, in the depression inferior to the spinous process of the seventh thoracic vertebra.

Acupuncture　Insert the needle obliquely 0.5~1.0 cun deep and stimulate until there is a sore and numbing sensation in the local area.

第一章 内科病证
Chapter 1 Medical diseases

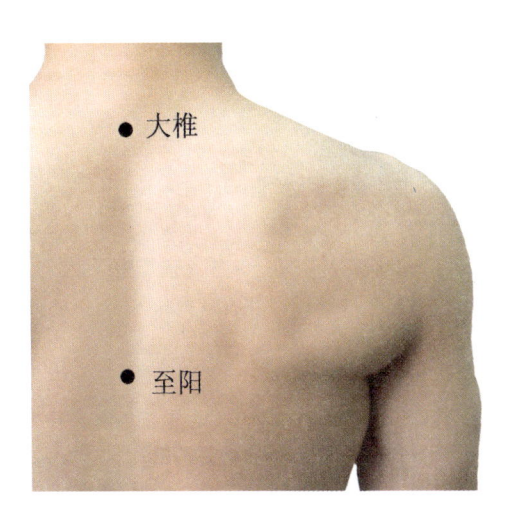

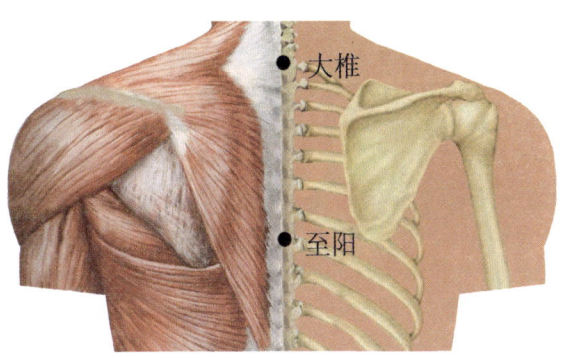

图1-12 大椎—至阳

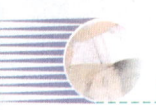

第十三节 水 肿

组合穴 中极—水道。

功 能 通利水道,利水消肿。

中极

【标准定位】在下腹部,脐中下4寸,前正中线上。

【毫针刺法】需排尿后进行针刺。直刺0.5~1.0寸,局部酸胀,可放射至外生殖器和会阴部。

水道

【标准定位】在下腹部,脐中下3寸,前正中线旁开2寸。

【毫针刺法】直刺0.5~1.0寸,局部酸胀。

Section 13　Edema

Combination Point 　Zhōng Jí—Shuǐdào.

Actions　Regulating fluid passage and treats edema.

RN 3　Zhōng Jí

Position　On the lower abdomen, on the anterior midline, 4 cun inferior to the umbilicus.

Acupuncture　Insert the needle after the micturition, perpendicularly 0.5~1.0 cun deep and stimulate until there is a sore and distending sensation in the local area radiating to the genitalia.

ST 28　Shuǐdào

Position　On the lower abdomen, 3 cun inferior to the umbilicus, 2 cun lateral to the anterior midline.

Acupuncture　Insert the needle perpendicularly 0.5~1.0 cun deep and stimulate until there is a sore and distending sensation in the local area.

第一章 内科病证
Chapter 1 Medical diseases

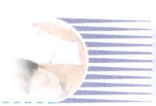

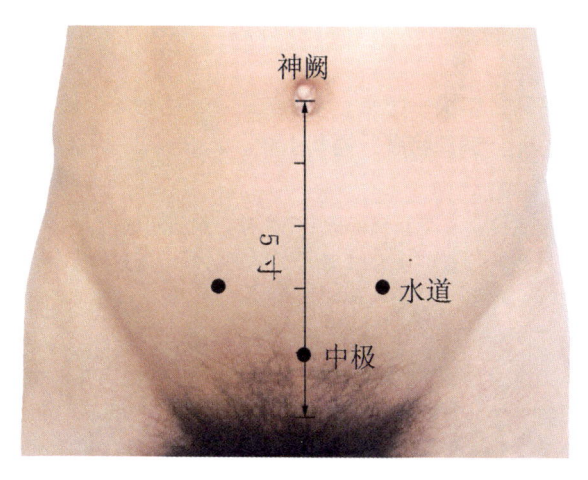

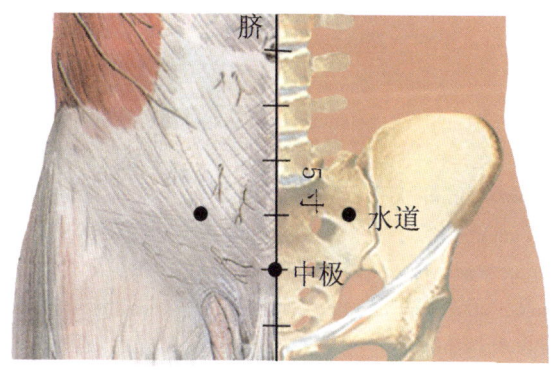

图1-13 中极—水道

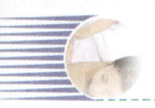

第十四节 癃 闭

组合穴 中极—归来。

功 能 调理膀胱，通利小便。

中极

【标准定位】 在下腹部，脐中下4寸，前正中线上。

【毫针刺法】 直刺0.5～1.0寸，局部酸胀，可放射至外生殖器和会阴部。

归来

【标准定位】 在下腹部，脐中下4寸，前下中线旁开2寸。

【毫针刺法】 直刺0.5～1.0寸，局部酸胀。

Section 14 Retention of urine

Combination Point Zhōng Jí—Guī Lái.

Actions Benefiting thebladder and inducing diuresis.

RN 3 Zhōng Jí.

Position On the lower abdomen, on the anterior midline, 4 cun inferior to the umbilicus.

Acupuncture Insert the needle perpendicularly 0.5～1.0 cun deep and stimulate until there is a sore and distending sensation in the local area radiating to the genitalia.

ST 29 Guī Lái

Position On the lower abdomen, 4 cun inferior to the umbilicus, 2 cun lateral from the anterior midline.

Acupuncture Insert the needle perpendicularly 0.5～1.0 cun deep and stimulate until there is a sore and distending sensation in the local area.

图 1-14 中极—归来

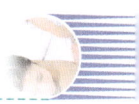

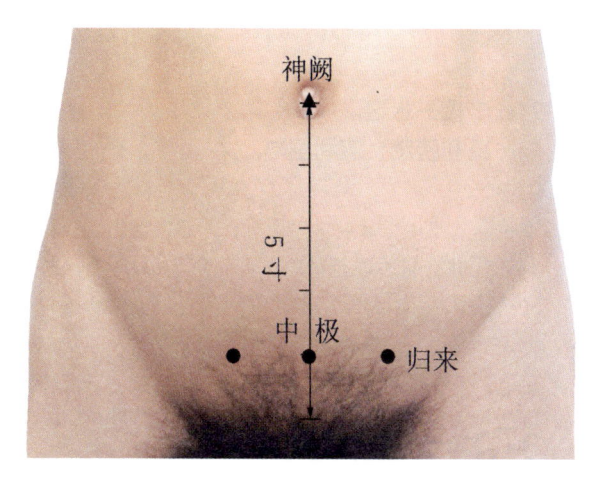

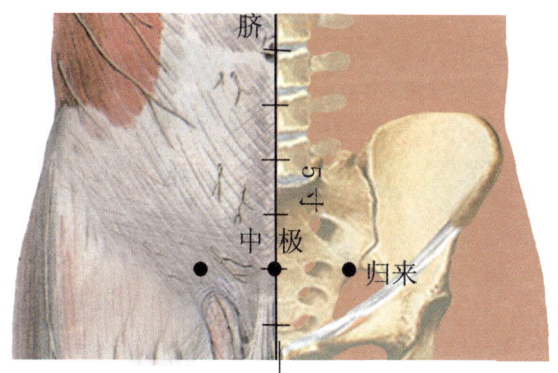

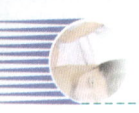

第十五节 淋 证

组合穴 中极—水道。

功 能 疏利膀胱,清利湿热。

中极

【标准定位】在下腹部,脐中下 4 寸,前正中线上。

【毫针刺法】需排尿后进行针刺。直刺 0.5~1.0 寸,局部酸胀,可放射至外生殖器和会阴部。

水道

【标准定位】在下腹部,脐中下 3 寸,前正中线旁开 2 寸。

【毫针刺法】直刺 0.5~1.0 寸,局部酸胀。

Section 15   Drench card

Combination Point   Zhōng Jí—Shuǐdào.

Actions   Dredging and benefiting the Bladder, transforming dampness and clearing heat.

RN 3 Zhōng Jí

Position   On the lower abdomen, on the anterior midline, 4 cun inferior to the umbilicus.

Acupuncture   Insert the needle after the micturition, perpendicularly 0.5~1.0 cun deep and stimulate until there is a sore and distending sensation in the local area radiating to the genitalia.

ST 28   Shuǐdào

Position   On the lower abdomen, 3 cun inferior to the umbilicus, 2 cun lateral to the anterior midline.

Acupuncture   Insert the needle perpendicularly 0.5~1.0 cun deep and stimulate until there is a sore and distending sensation in the local area.

图1-15 中极—水道

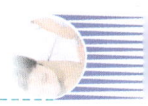

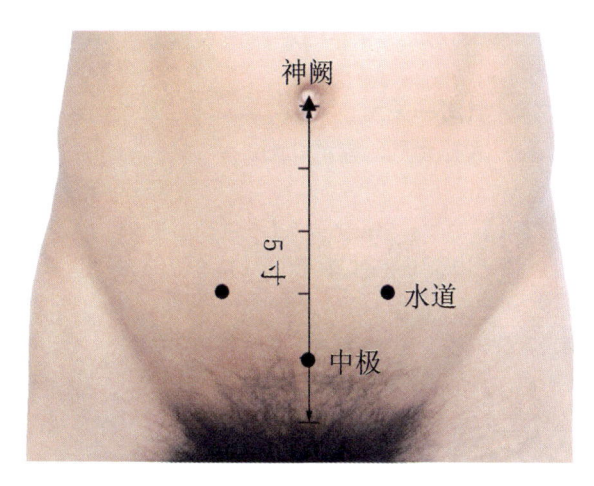

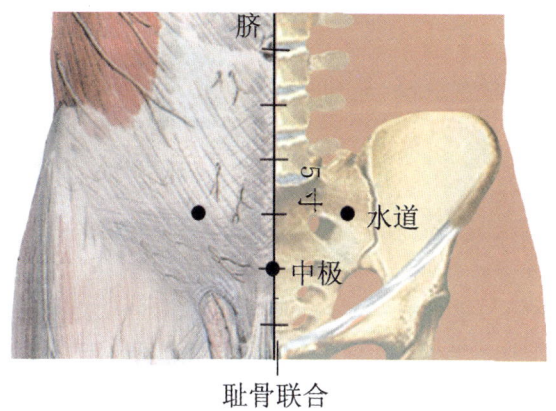

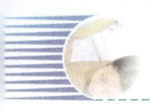

第十六节 尿失禁

组合穴 气海—关元。

功　能 大补元气，温肾助阳。

气海

【标准定位】在下腹部，脐中下 1.5 寸，前正中线上。

【毫针刺法】直刺 0.8～1.2 寸，局部酸胀。

关元

【标准定位】在下腹部，脐中下 3 寸，前正中线上。

【毫针刺法】需排尿后进行针刺。直刺 0.5～1.0 寸，局部酸胀，可放射至外生殖器和会阴部。

Section 16　Urinary incontinence

Combination Point　Qì Hǎi—Guān Yuán.

Actions　Tonifying original qi and benefiting essence, tonifying kidney and fortifying yang.

RN 6 Qì Hǎi

Position　On the lower abdomen, on the anterior midline, 1.5 cun inferior to the umbilicus.

Acupuncture　Insert the needle perpendicularly 0.8～1.2 cun deep and stimulate until there is a sore and distending sensation in the local area.

RN4 Guān Yuán

Position　On the lower abdomen, on the anterior midline, 3 cun inferior to the umbilicus.

Acupuncture　Insert the needle after the micturition, perpendicularly 0.5～1.0 cun deep and stimulate until there is a sore and distending sensation in the local area radiating to the genitalia.

图 1-16 气海—关元

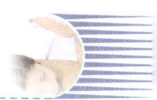

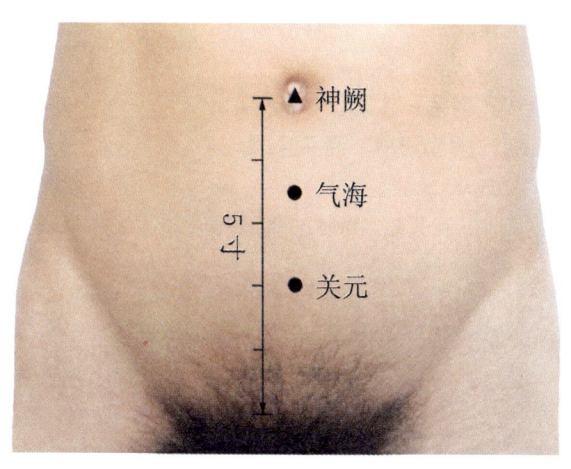

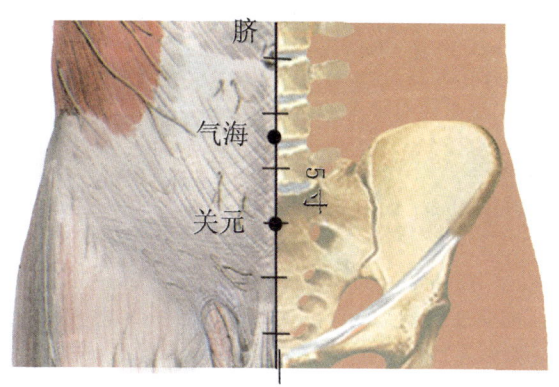

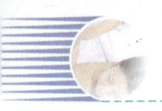

第十七节　头　痛

组合穴　百会—太阳。

功　能　镇惊安神，清头止痛。

百会

【标准定位】在头部，当前发际正中直上5寸，或两耳尖连线的中点处。

【毫针刺法】平刺，针尖可向四周进针0.5～0.8寸。

太阳

【标准定位】在头部，眉梢与目外眦之间，向后约一横指的凹陷中。

【毫针刺法】直刺0.3～0.5寸，局部酸胀；或向后平刺1.0～2.0寸，透率谷，局部酸胀。

Section 17　Headache

Combination Point　Bǎi Huì—Tài Yáng.

Actions　Calming the spirit, clearing the head and alleviating pain.

DU 20 Bǎi Huì

Position　On the head, 5 cun posterior to the midpoint of the anterior hairline, and at the midpoint of the line between the two ears.

Acupuncture　Insert the needle subcutaneously 0.5～0.8 cun deep.

EX–HN 5 Tài Yáng

Position　In the depression about one finger breadth posterior to the midpoint between the lateral end of the eyebrow and the outer canthus.

Acupuncture　Insert the needle perpendicularly 0.3～0.5 cun deep and stimulate until there is a sore and distending sensation in the local area.

第一章 内科病证
Chapter 1　Medical diseases

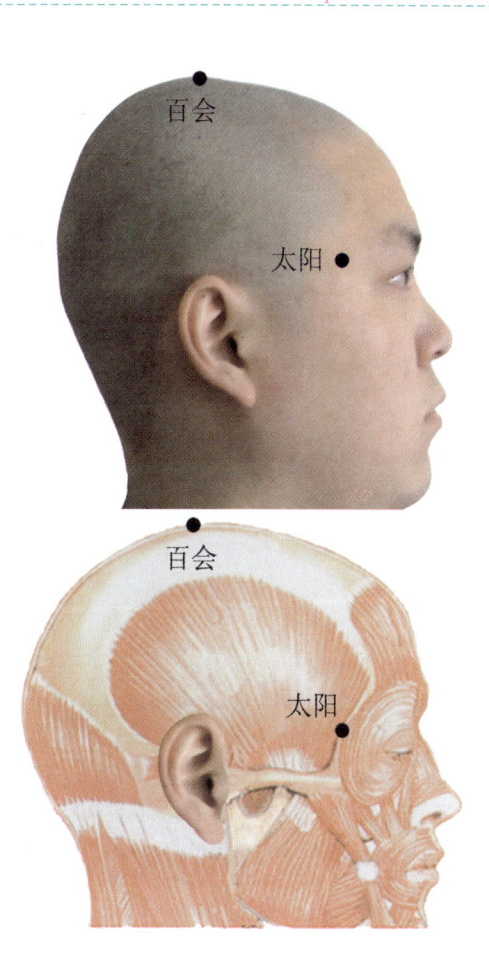

百会

太阳

百会

太阳

图1-17　百会—太阳

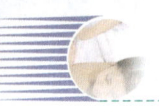

第十八节 三叉神经痛

组合穴 太阳—下关。
功 能 通络止痛。

太阳

【标准定位】在头部,眉梢与目外眦之间,向后约一横指的凹陷中。

【毫针刺法】直刺 0.3~0.5 寸,局部酸胀;或向后平刺 1.0~2.0 寸,透率谷。

下关

【标准定位】当颧弓与下颌切迹所形成的凹陷处。

【毫针刺法】直刺 0.8~1.2 寸。

Section 18　Trigeminal neuralgia

Combination Point　Tài Yáng—Xià Guān.

Actions　Activating the channel and alleviating pain.

EX – HN 5 Tài Yáng

Position　In the depression about one finger breadth posterior to the midpoint between the lateral end of the eyebrow and the outer canthus.

AcupunctureInsert the needle perpendicularly 0.3~0.5 cun deep and penetrate to GB 8 (Shuài Gǔ).

ST 7 Xià Guān

Position　In the depression between the zygomatic arch and mandibular notch in front of the ear.

Acupuncture　Insert the needle perpendicularly 0.8~1.2 cun deep.

图1-18　太阳—下关

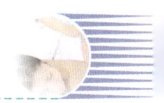

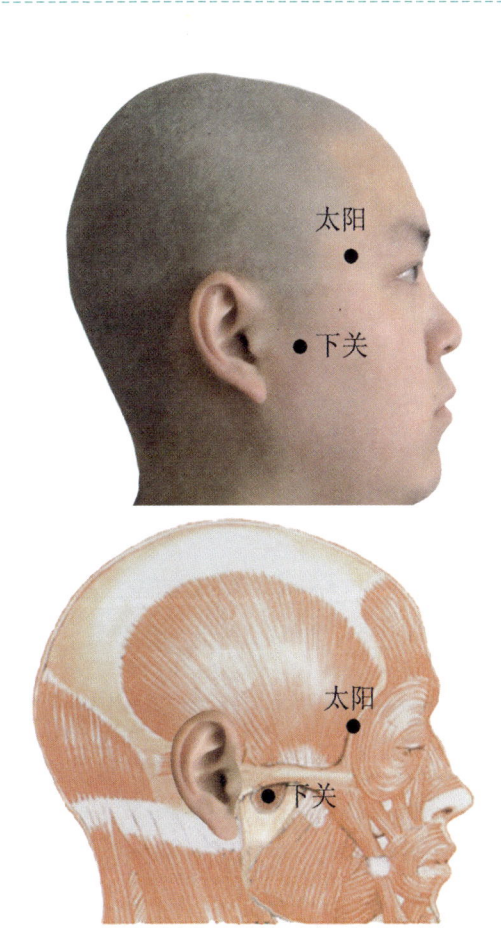

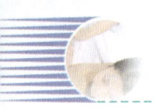

第十九节 面 瘫

组合穴 地仓—颊车。
功 能 祛风通络。

地仓
【标准定位】在面部,当口角旁开0.4寸。
【毫针刺法】向颊车方向平刺1.0~2.5寸,局部酸胀。

颊车
【标准定位】在面部,下颌角前上方一横指(中指)。
【毫针刺法】平刺1.0~2.0寸透地仓穴。

Section 19 Facial paralysis

Combination Point Dì Cāng—Jiá Chē.

Actions Expelling wind and activating the collaterals.

ST 4 Dì Cāng

Position On the face, directly inferior to ST 3 (jù liáo) at the level with the corner of the mouth.

Acupuncture Insert the needle subcutaneously towards ST 6 (Jiá Chē) 1.0~2.5 cun deep and stimulate until there is a sore and numbing sensation in the local area.

ST 6 Jiá Chē

Position On the cheek, in the depression one finger-breadth anterior and superior to the corner of the mandible, on the prominence of the muscle when the teeth are clenched.

Acupuncture Insert the needle subcutaneously towards ST 4 (Dì Cāng) 0.5~0.8 cun deep.

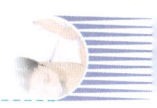

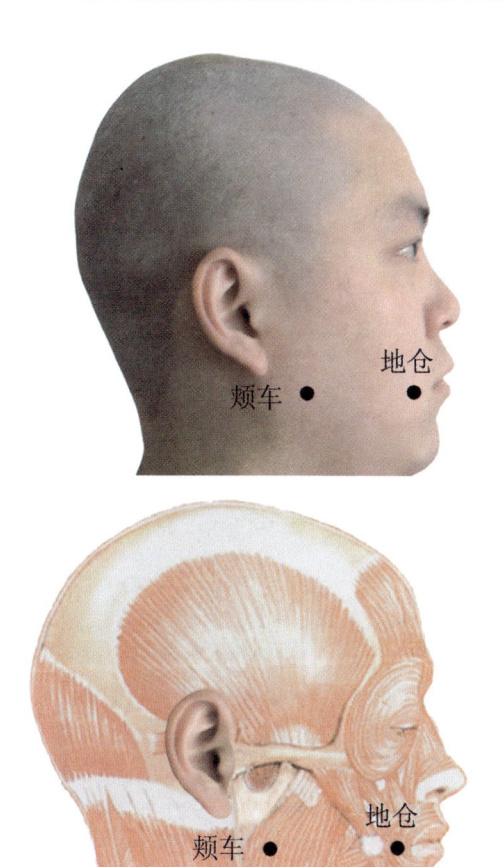

图1-19 地仓—颊车

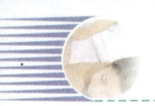

第二十节　面肌痉挛

组合穴　太阳—四白。

功　能　平肝熄风，通络止痉。

太阳

【标准定位】在头部，眉梢与目外眦之间，向后约一横指的凹陷中。

【毫针刺法】直刺 0.3~0.5 寸，局部酸胀；或向后平刺 1.0~2.0 寸，透率谷。

四白

【标准定位】在面部，眶下孔处。

【毫针刺法】直刺 0.3~0.5 寸，局部酸胀。

Section 20　Hemifacial spasm

Combination Point　Tài Yáng—Sì Bái.

Actions　Calming the liver to stop the wind, activating the collaterals and alleviating pain spasm.

EX–HN 5 Tài Yáng

Position　In the depression about one finger breadth posterior to the midpoint between the lateral end of the eyebrow and the outer canthus.

AcupunctureInsert the needle perpendicularly 0.3~0.5 cun deep and penetrate to GB 8 (Shuài Gǔ).

ST 2 Sì Bái

Position　On the face, inferior to the pupil in the depression of the infraorbital foramen.

Acupuncture　Insert the needle perpendicularly 0.3~0.5cun deep until there is a soreness and numbness sensation in the local area.

第一章　内科病证

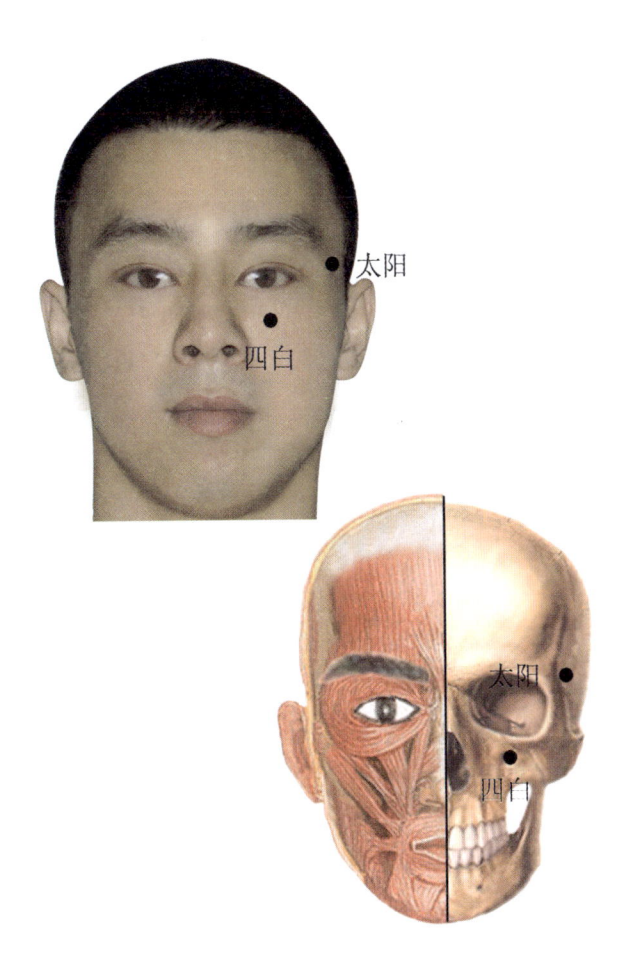

Chapter 1　Medical diseases

图1-20　太阳—四白

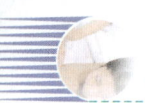

第二十一节 眩 晕

组合穴 风池—太阳。

功 能 清利头目,安神止眩。

风池

【标准定位】在颈后区,胸锁乳突肌上端与斜方肌上端之间的凹陷中。

【毫针刺法】向鼻尖方向斜刺 0.5~1.5 寸。

太阳

【标准定位】在头部,眉梢与目外眦之间,向后约一横指的凹陷中。

【毫针刺法】直刺 0.3~0.5 寸,局部酸胀。

Section 21　Vertigo

Combination Point　Fēng Chí—Tài Yáng.

Actions　Clearing the head and eyes, Calming the spirit and alleviating vertigo.

GB20 Fēng Chí

Position　On the nape, in the depression between m. sternocleidomastoideus and m. trapezius.

Acupuncture　Insert the needle obliquely toward the apex nasi 0.5~1.5 cun deep.

EX–HN 5 Tài Yáng

Position　In the depression about one finger breadth posterior to the midpoint between the lateral end of the eyebrow and the outer canthus.

Acupuncture　Insert the needle perpendicularly 0.3~0.5 cun deep and stimulate until there is a sore and distending sensation in the local area.

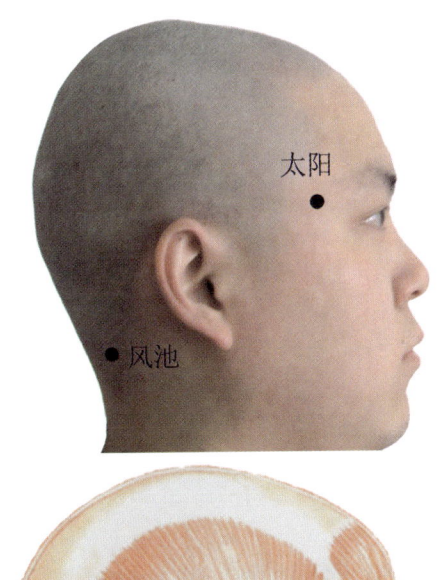

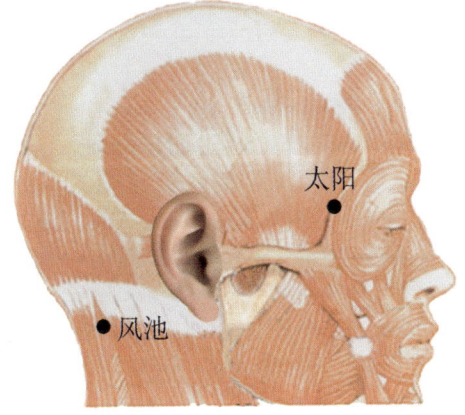

图1-21 风池—太阳

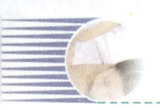

第二十二节 高血压病

组合穴 合谷—太冲。

功 能 平肝潜阳。

合谷

【标准定位】在手背,第1、2掌骨间,第2掌骨桡侧的中点处。

【毫针刺法】直刺0.5~1.0寸。

太冲

【标准定位】在足背,当第1、2跖骨间,跖骨底结合部前方凹陷中。

【毫针刺法】向上斜刺0.5~1.0,局部酸胀。

Section 22 Hypertensive disease

Combination Point Hé Gǔ—Tài Chōng.

Actions Spreading Liver qi and Subdues Liver yang.

LI 4 Hé Gǔ

Position On the dorsum of the hand, between the first and second metacarpal bones, on the radial side of the middle of the second metacarpal bone.

Acupuncture Insert the needle perpendicularly 0.5~1.0 cun deep.

LV 3 Tài Chōng

Position On the dorsum of the foot, in the depression proximal to the first metatarsal space.

Acupuncture Insert the needle obliquely upwards 0.5~1.0 cun deep and stimulate until there is a sore and numbing sensation.

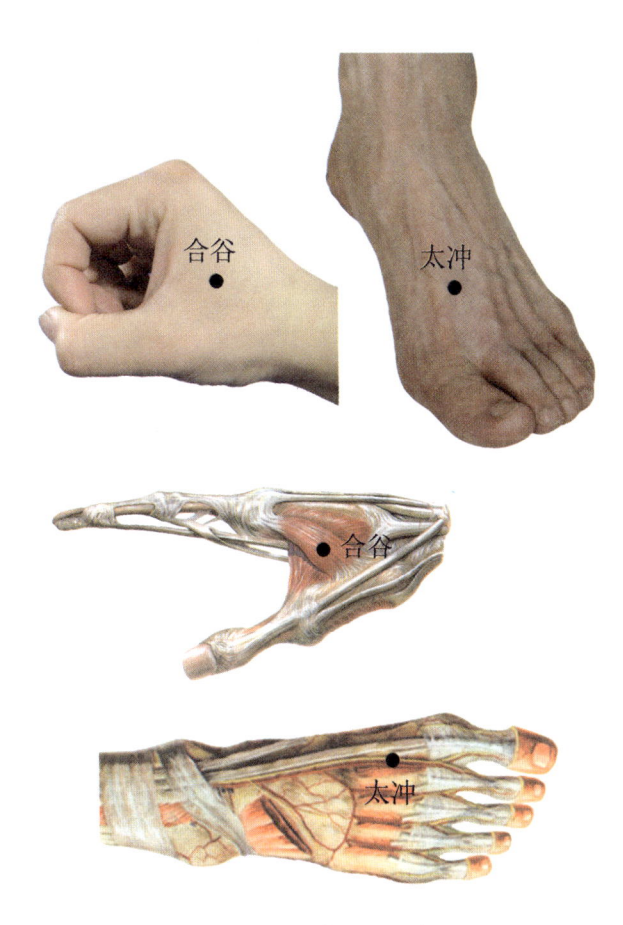

图 1-22 合谷—太冲

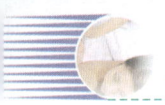

第二十三节 低血压

组合穴 百会—足三里。
功　能 健脾益气。

百会
【标准定位】在头部,当前发际正中直上5寸,或两耳尖连线的中点处。
【毫针刺法】平刺,针尖可向四周进针0.5~0.8寸。

足三里
【标准定位】在小腿外侧,犊鼻(ST 35)下3寸,犊鼻(ST 35)与解溪(ST 41)连线上。
【毫针刺法】直刺0.5~1.5寸,局部酸胀。

Section 23　Hypotension

Combination Point　Bǎi Huì— Shén Tíng.

Actions　Invigorating the Spleen and tonifying qi.

DU 20 Bǎi Huì

Position　On the head, 5 cun posterior to the midpoint of the anterior hairline, and at the midpoint of the line between the two ears.

Acupuncture　Insert the needle subcutaneously 0.5~0.8 cun deep.

ST36 Zú Sān Lǐ

Position　On the anterior aspect of the lower leg, 3 cun distal to ST 35 (dú bí), one finger width lateral from the anterior ridge of the tibia.

Acupuncture　Insert the needle perpendicularly 0.5~1.5 cun deep and stimulate until there is a sore and distending sensation.

第一章 内科病证
Chapter 1　Medical diseases

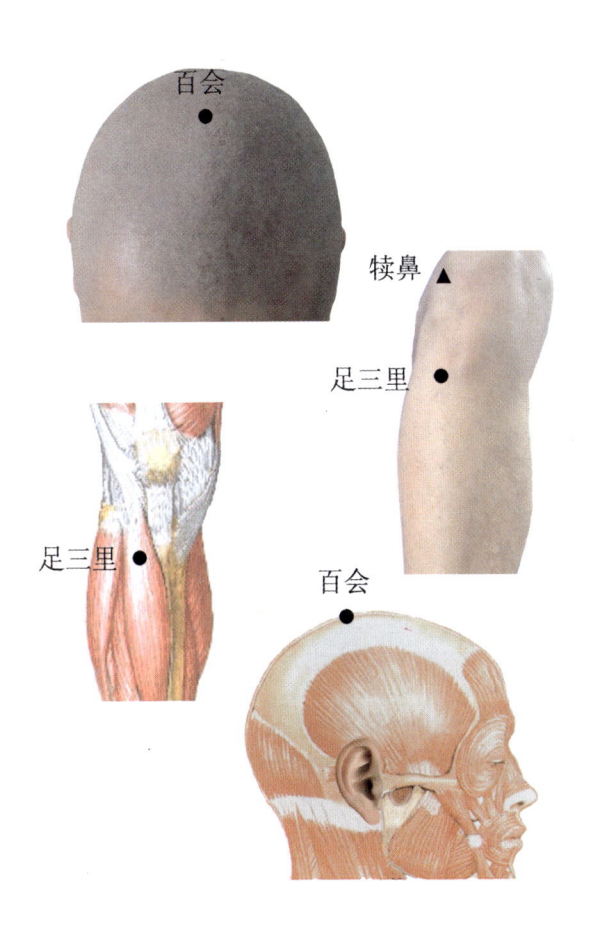

图1-23　百会—足三里

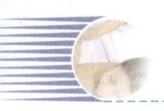

第二十四节 贫 血

组合穴 足三里—三阴交。
功 能 益气养血。

足三里

【标准定位】在小腿外侧,犊鼻(ST 35)下3寸,犊鼻(ST 35)与解溪(ST 41)连线上。

【毫针刺法】直刺0.5~1.5寸,局部酸胀。

三阴交

【标准定位】当足内踝尖上3寸,胫骨内侧缘后方。

【毫针刺法】直刺1.0~1.5寸。孕妇不宜针。

Section 24 Anemia

Combination Point Zú Sān Lǐ—Sān Yīn Jiāo.

Actions Tonifying qi and nourishing blood.

ST36 Zú Sān Lǐ

Position On the anterior aspect of the lower leg, 3 cun distal to ST 35 (dú bí), one finger width lateral from the anterior ridge of the tibia.

Acupuncture Insert the needle perpendicularly 0.5~1.5 cun deep and stimulate until there is a sore and distending sensation.

SP 6 Sān Yīn Jiāo

Position On the medial part of the leg, 3 cun superior to the tip of medial malleolus, posterior to the medial edge of the tibia.

Acupuncture Insert the needle perpendicularly 0.5~1.5 cun deep and stimulate until there is a sore and numbing sensation in the local area.

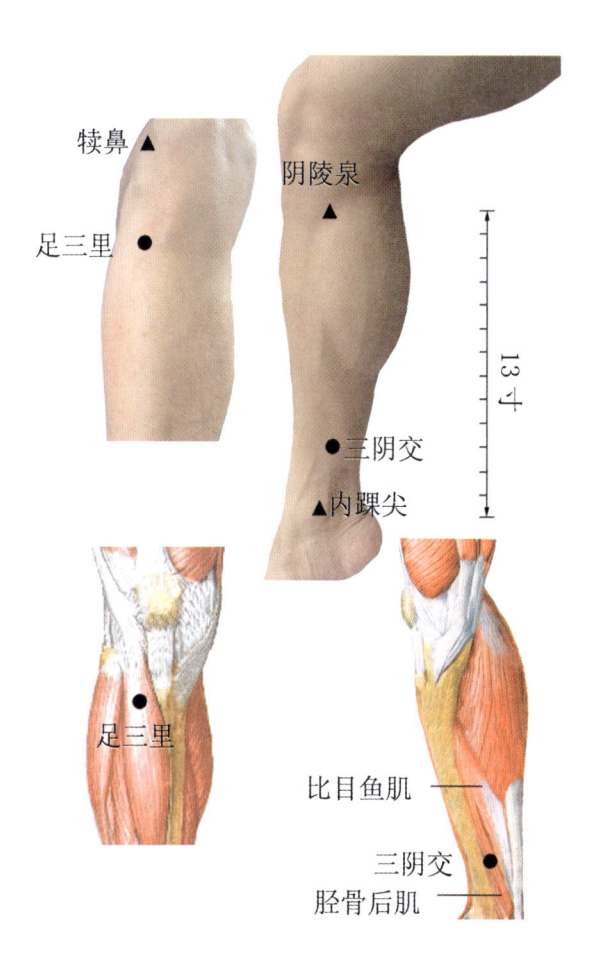

图1-24　足三里—三阴交

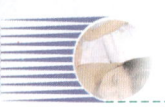

第二十五节 心 悸

组合穴 内关—膻中。

功 能 宽胸理气,宁心定悸。

内关

【标准定位】在前臂前区,腕掌侧远端横纹上2寸,掌长肌腱与桡侧腕屈肌腱之间。

【毫针刺法】直刺0.5~1.0寸。

膻中

【标准定位】在胸部,当前正中线上,平第四肋间,两乳头连线的中点。

【毫针刺法】平刺0.3~0.5寸。

Section 25 Palpitations

Combination Point Nèi Guān—Tán Zhōng.

Actions Unbinding the chest and regulating qi, calming spirit and alleviating palpitations.

PC 6 Nèi Guān

Position On the palmar aspect of the forearm, 2 cun superior to the transverse crease of the wrist, between palmaris longus tendon and flexor carpi radialis tendon.

Acupuncture Insert the needle perpendicularly 0.5~1.0 cun deep.

RN17 Tán Zhōng

Position On the chest, on the anterior midline, at the level of the fourth intercostal space, at the midpoint between the two nipples.

Acupuncture Insert the needle subcutaneously or obliquely 0.3~0.5 cun deep.

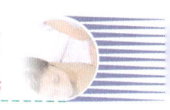

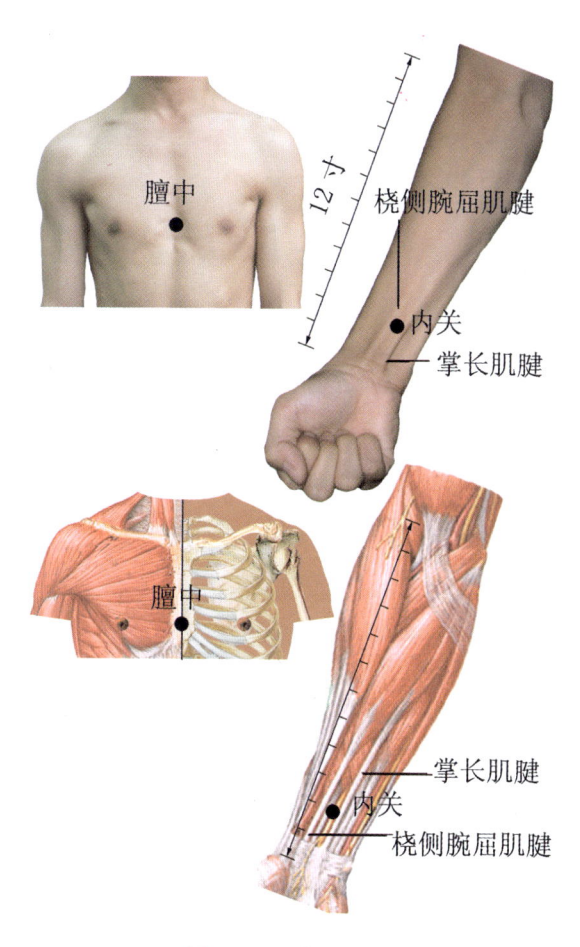

图1-25 内关—膻中

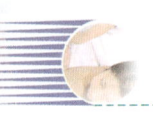

第二十六节 失 眠

组合穴 内关—三阴交。
功 能 宁心安神。

内关
【标准定位】在前臂前区，腕掌侧远端横纹上 2 寸，掌长肌腱与桡侧腕屈肌腱之间。
【毫针刺法】直刺 0.5～1.5 寸，局部酸胀。

三阴交
【标准定位】当足内踝尖上 3 寸，胫骨内侧缘后方。
【毫针刺法】直刺 1.0～1.5 寸。孕妇不宜针。

Section 26 Insomnia

Combination Point Nèi Guān—Sān Yīn Jiāo.

Actions Calming the heart and spirit.

PC 6 Nèi Guān

Position On the palmar aspect of the forearm, 2 cun superior to the transverse crease of the wrist, between palmaris longus tendon and flexor carpi radialis tendon.

Acupuncture Insert the needle perpendicularly 0.5～1.5 cun deep and stimulate until there is a sore and numbing sensation.

SP 6 Sān Yīn Jiāo

Position On the medial part of the leg, 3 cun superior to the tip of medial malleolus, posterior to the medial edge of the tibia.

Acupuncture Insert the needle perpendicularly 0.5～1.5 cun deep and stimulate until there is a sore and numbing sensation in the local area.

第一章　内科病证
Chapter 1　Medical diseases

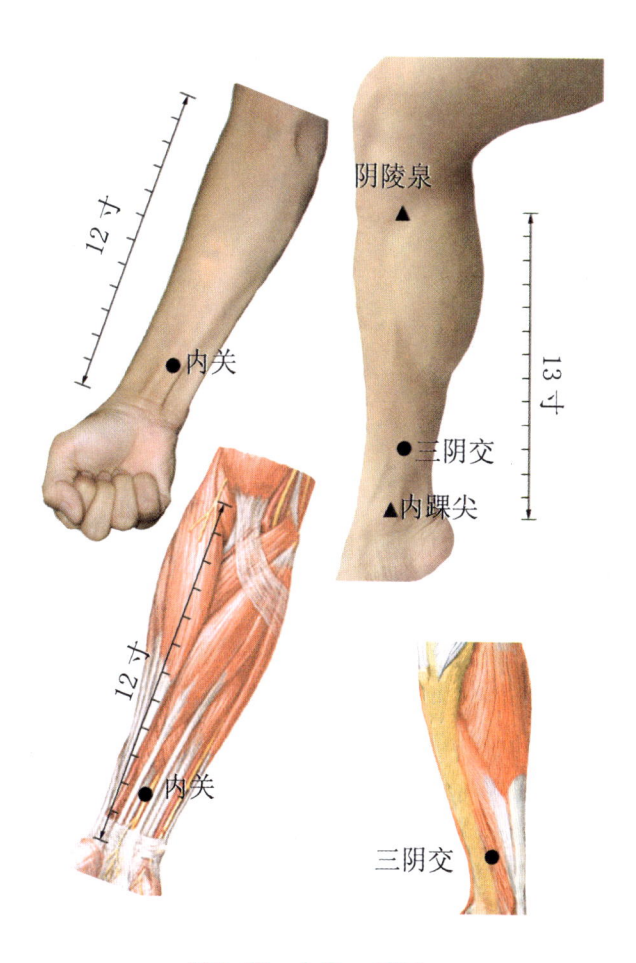

图 1-26　内关—三阴交

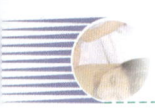

第二十七节 痴 呆

组合穴 百会—神门。
功 能 开窍益智。

百会

【标准定位】在头部,当前发际正中直上 5 寸,或两耳尖连线的中点处。

【毫针刺法】平刺,针尖可向四周进针 0.5~0.8 寸。

神门

【标准定位】在腕前区,腕掌侧远端横纹尺侧端,尺侧腕屈肌腱的桡侧缘。

【毫针刺法】平刺 0.3~0.5 寸,局部胀痛。

Section 27   Dementia

Combination Point   Bǎi Huì— Shén Tíng.

Actions   activiting brain and regaining consciousness.

DU 20 Bǎi Huì

Position   On the head, 5 cun posterior to the midpoint of the anterior hairline, and at the midpoint of the line between the two ears.

Acupuncture   Insert the needle subcutaneously 0.5~0.8 cun deep.

HT 7   Shénmén

Position   On the radial side of the tendon m. flexor carpi ulnaris of the transverse wrist crease.

Acupuncture   Insert the needle perpendicularly 0.3~0.5 cun deep.

第一章 内科病证
Chapter 1 Medical diseases

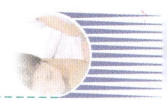

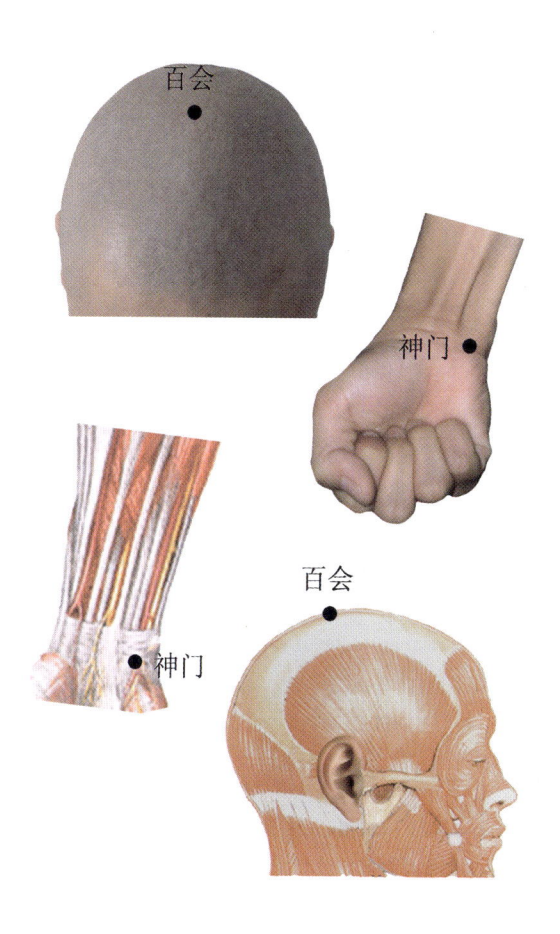

图1-27 百会—神门

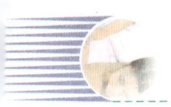

第二十八节 癫 病

组合穴 心俞—神门。

功 能 养心开窍醒神。

心俞

【标准定位】第5胸椎棘突下,后正中线旁开1.5寸。

【毫针刺法】向内斜刺0.5~0.8寸,局部酸胀。

神门

【标准定位】在腕前区,腕掌侧远端横纹尺侧端,尺侧腕屈肌腱的桡侧缘。

【毫针刺法】平刺0.3~0.5寸,局部胀痛。

Section 28　Depressive psychosis

Combination Point　Xīn Shū—Shénmén.

Actions　Nourishing the heart and activiting spirit.

BL 15　Xīn Shū

Position　On the upper back, 1.5 cun lateral to the lower border of the spinous process of the fifth thoracic vertebra.

Acupuncture　Insert the needle obliquely towards the spine 0.5~0.8 cun deep and stimulate until there is a sore and numbing sensation.

HT 7　Shénmén

Position　On the radial side of the tendon m. flexor carpi ulnaris of the transverse wrist crease.

Acupuncture　Insert the needle perpendicularly 0.3~0.5 cun deep.

第一章 内科病证
Chapter 1 Medical diseases

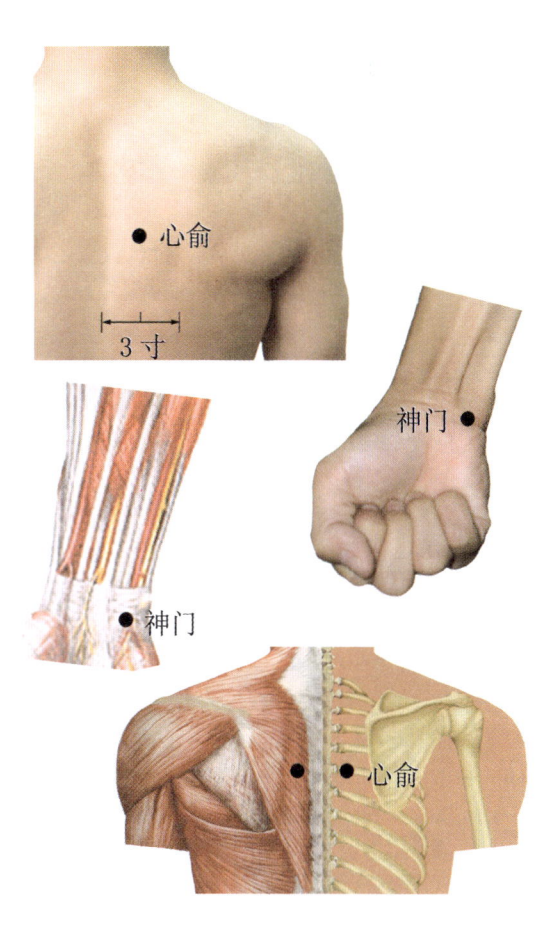

图 1-28 心俞—神门

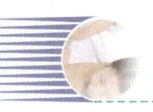

第二十九节 痫 病

组合穴　水沟—内关。

功　能　开窍醒神、定惊止痫。

水沟

【标准定位】在面部，人中沟的上 1/3 与中 1/3 交点处。

【毫针刺法】向上斜刺 0.2~0.3 寸，局部酸胀。

内关

【标准定位】在前臂前区，腕掌侧远端横纹上 2 寸，掌长肌腱与桡侧腕屈肌腱之间。

【毫针刺法】直刺 0.5~1.5 寸，局部酸胀。

Section 29　Epilepsy

Combination Point　Shuǐ Gōu—Nèi Guān.

Actions　Activiting brain and regaining consciousness, Calming the spirit and alleviating epilepsy.

DU 26　Shuǐ Gōu

Position　On the face, at the junction of the superior 1/3 and inferior 2/3 of the philtrum.

Acupuncture　Insert the needle obliquely upwards 0.2~0.3 cun deep and stimulate until there is a sore and numbing sensation in the local area.

PC 6 Nèi Guān

Position　On the palmar aspect of the forearm, 2 cun superior to the transverse crease of the wrist, between palmaris longus tendon and flexor carpi radialis tendon.

Acupuncture　Insert the needle perpendicularly 0.5~1.5 cun deep and stimulate until there is a sore and numbing sensation.

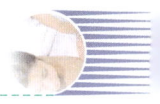

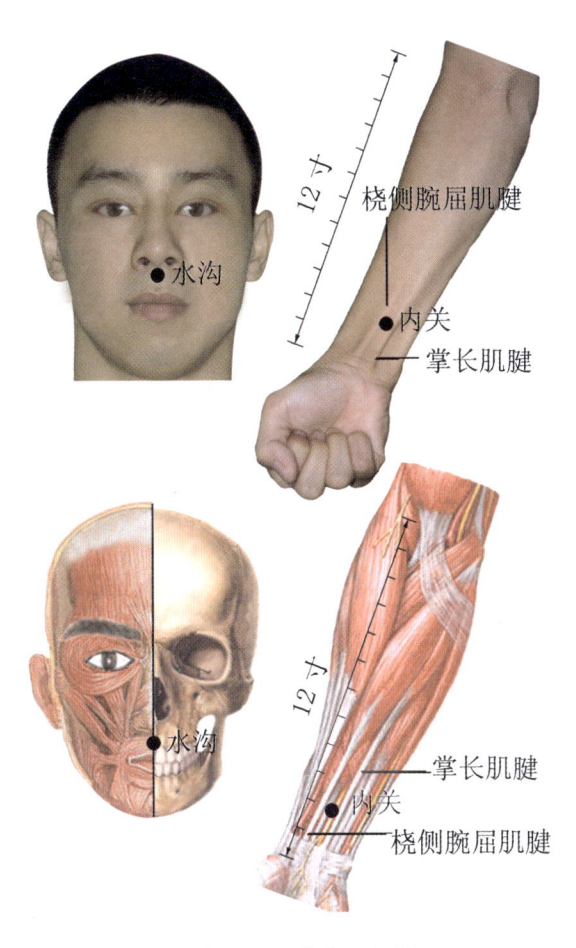

图1-29 水沟—内关

第三十节 癔病

组合穴 合谷—太冲。

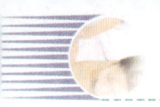

功 能 条畅气机。

合谷

【标准定位】在手背,第1、2掌骨间,第2掌骨桡侧的中点处。

【毫针刺法】直刺0.5~1.0寸,局部酸胀。

太冲

【标准定位】在足背,当第1、2跖骨间,跖骨底结合部前方凹陷中。

【毫针刺法】向上斜刺0.5~1.0寸,局部酸胀。

Section 30 Hysteria

Combination Point Hé Gǔ—Tài Chōng.

Actions Regulating and smoothing qi.

LI 4 Hé Gǔ

Position On the dorsum of the hand, between the first and second metacarpal bones, on the radial side of the middle of the second metacarpal bone.

Acupuncture Insert the needle perpendicularly 0.5~1.0 cun deep.

LV 3 Tài Chōng

Position On the dorsum of the foot, in the depression proximal to the first metatarsal space.

Acupuncture Insert the needle obliquely upwards 0.5~1.0 cun deep and stimulate until there is a sore and numbing sensation.

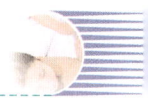

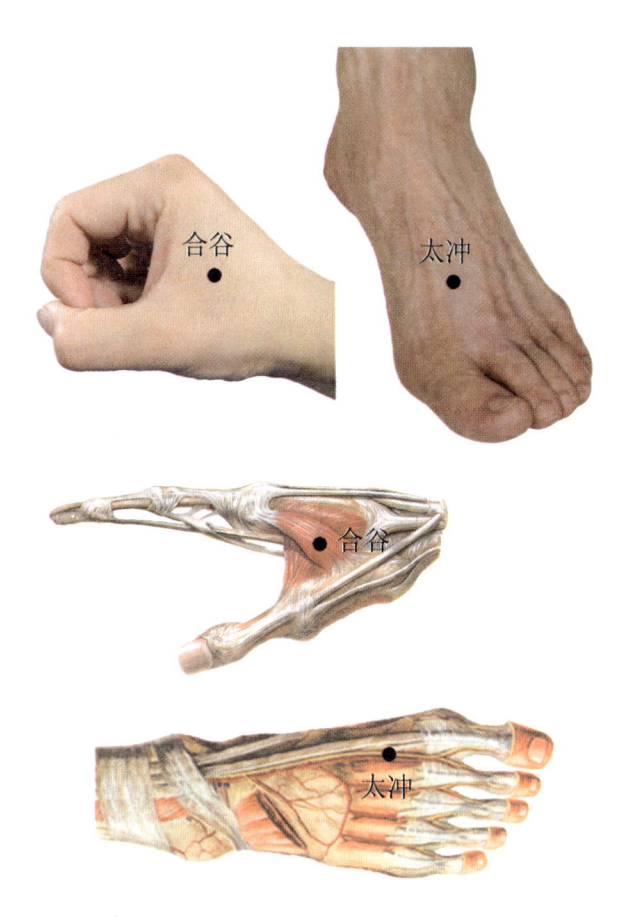

图1-30　合谷—太冲

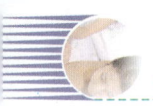

第三十一节 震颤麻痹

组合穴 风池—太冲。
功 能 平肝熄风止痉。

风池
【标准定位】在颈后区,胸锁乳突肌上端与斜方肌上端之间的凹陷中。
【毫针刺法】向鼻尖方向斜刺 0.5~1.5 寸。

太冲
【标准定位】在足背,当第 1、2 跖骨间,跖骨底结合部前方凹陷中。
【毫针刺法】向上斜刺 0.5~1.0,局部酸胀。

Section 31 Paralysis agitans

Combination Point Fēng Chí—Tài Chōng.

Actions Calming the liver to stop the wind and alleviating spasm.

GB20 Fēng Chí

Position On the nape, in the depression between m. sternocleidomastoideus and m. trapezius.

Acupuncture Insert the needle obliquely toward the apex nasi 0.5~1.5 cun deep.

LV 3 Tài Chōng

Position On the dorsum of the foot, in the depression proximal to the first metatarsal space.

Acupuncture Insert the needle obliquely upwards 0.5~1.0 cun deep and stimulate until there is a sore and numbing sensation.

第一章 内科病证
Chapter 1 Medical diseases

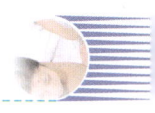

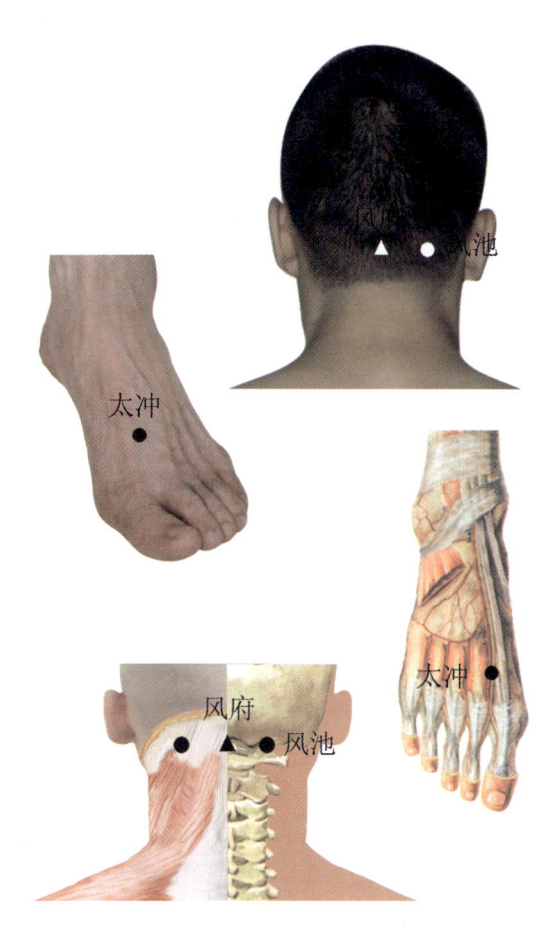

图 1-31 风池—太冲

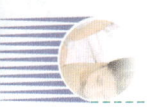

第三十二节 痹 证

1. 肩部

组合穴 肩髃—肩髎。

功 能 通利关节,祛风除湿。

肩髃

【标准定位】当肩峰与肱骨大结节之间凹陷处。

【毫针刺法】直刺 1~1.5 寸,局部酸胀。

肩髎

【标准定位】肩峰角与肱骨大结节两骨间凹陷中。

【毫针刺法】直刺 1~1.5 寸,局部酸胀。

Section 32 Arthralgia syndrome

1. Shoulder

Combination Point Jiān Yú— Jiān Liáo.

Actions Dispelling wind–dampness activating the channel and benefiting the joint.

LI 15 Jiān Yú

Position In the anterior and inferior aspect of the acromion, in the depression between the acromion and the greater tubercle of the humerus.

Acupuncture Insert the needle perpendicularly 1~1.5cun deep.

SJ 14 Jiān Liáo

Position On the shoulder, posterior to LI 15 (jiān yú), when the arm is abducted, in the depression posterior and inferior to the acromion.

Acupuncture Insert the needle perpendicularly 1~1.5 cun deep and stimulate until there is a sore and distending sensation.

肩髃●
肩髎●

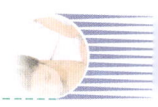

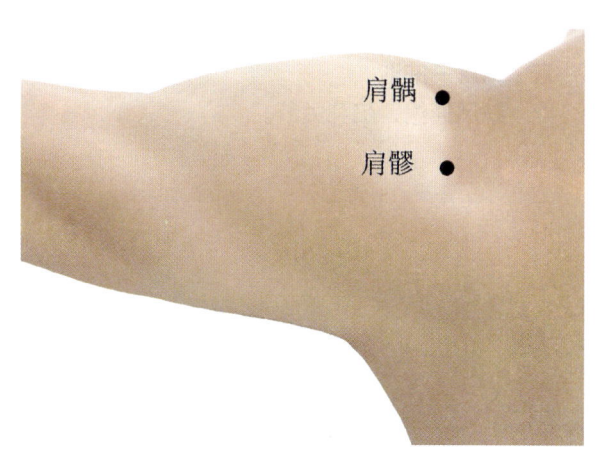

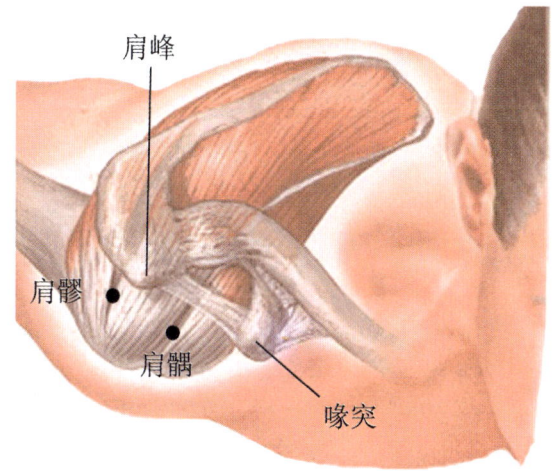

肩峰
肩髎●
肩髃●
喙突

图1-32-1 肩髃—肩髎

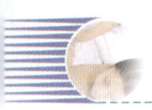

2. 肘部

组合穴 臂臑—曲池。

功 能 祛风通络，疏利关节。

臂臑

【标准定位】在臂部，曲池上7寸，三角肌前缘处。

【毫针刺法】直刺0.5~1寸。

曲池

【标准定位】在肘区，尺泽与肱骨外上髁上连线的中点处。

【毫针刺法】直刺1.0~2.0寸。

2. Elbow

Combination Point Bì Nào— Qǔ Chí.

Actions expelling wind and activating collaterals, benefiting the joint.

LI 14 Bì Nào

Position On the lateral side of the upper arm, 7 cun proximal to LI 11 (qǔ chí) on the line connecting LI 11 (qǔ chí) and LI 15 (jiān yú), in the depression formed by the distal insertion of the m. deltoideus and m. brachialis.

Acupuncture Insert the needle perpendicularly 0.5~1 cun deep.

LI 11 Qǔ Chí

Position In the depression of the radial side of the transverse cubital crease when elbow flexed.

Acupuncture Insert the needle perpendicularly 1.0~2.0 cun deep.

第一章 内科病证
Chapter 1　Medical diseases

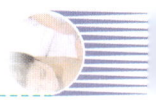

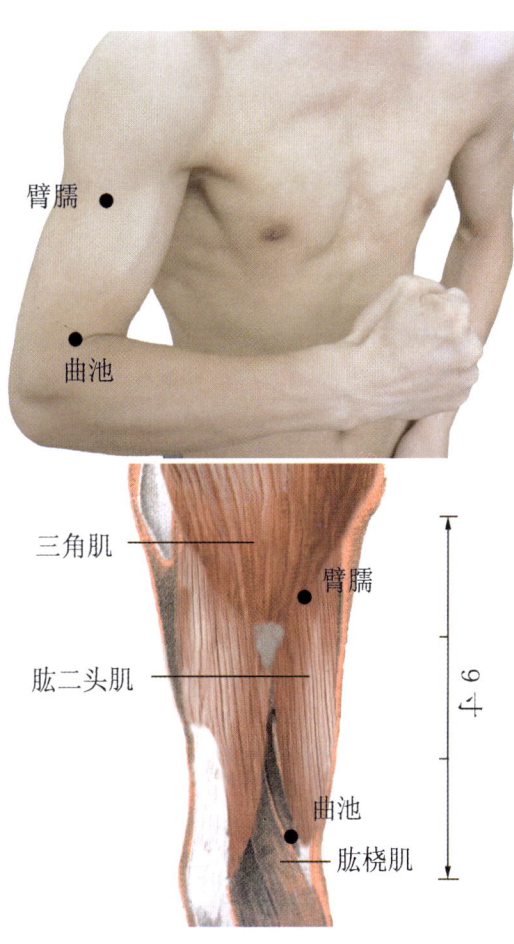

图 1-32-2　臂臑—曲池

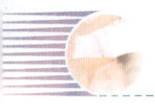

3. 腕部

组合穴　阳溪—阳谷。

功　能　清热散风，舒筋利节。

阳溪

【标准定位】 在腕区，腕背侧远端横纹桡侧，桡骨茎突远端，解剖学"鼻烟窝"凹陷中。

【毫针刺法】 直刺 0.5～0.8 寸。

阳谷

【标准定位】 在腕后区，尺骨茎突与三角骨之间的凹陷中。

【毫针刺法】 直刺 0.3～0.5 寸，局部酸胀，可扩散至整个腕关节。

3. Wrist

Combination Point　Yáng Xī— Yáng Gǔ.

Actions　Expelling wind Clearing heat, activating collaterals.

LI 5 Yáng Xī

Position　On the dorsal side of the wrist, in the depression between the tendons of m. extensor pollicis longus and m. extensor pollicis brevis.

Acupuncture　Insert the needle perpendicularly 0.5～0.8 cun deep.

SI 5 Yáng Gǔ

Position　On the ulnar side of the wrist, in the depression between the styloid process of the ulna and the triangular bone.

Acupuncture　Insert the needle perpendicularly 0.3～0.5 cun deep and stimulate until there is a sore and numbing sensation in the local area radiating in the wrist.

第一章 内科病证
Chapter 1 Medical diseases

阳溪 ● ● 阳谷

阳溪

阳谷

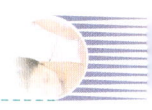

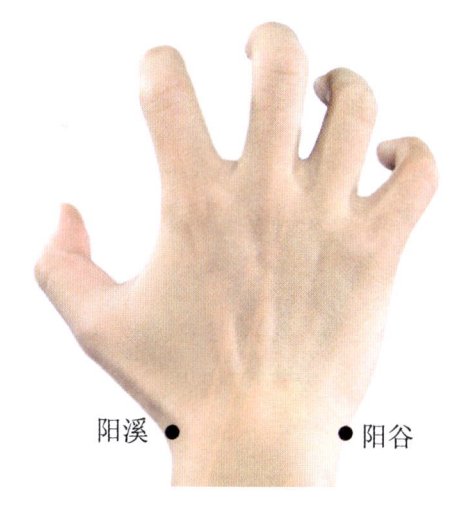

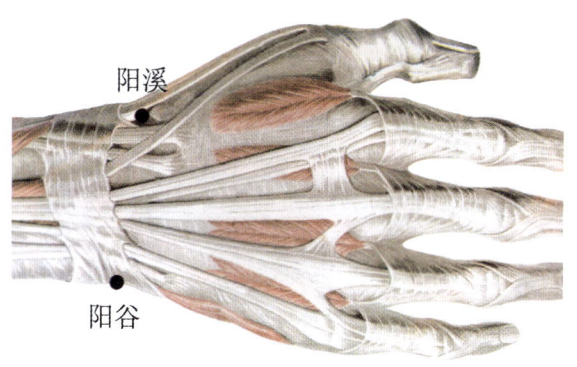

图 1-32-3 阳溪—阳谷

4. 脊背

组合穴 大椎—至阳。

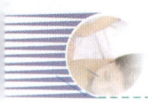

功　能 祛风解表，利胆退黄。

大椎

【标准定位】在脊柱区，第 7 颈椎棘突下凹陷中，后正中线上。

【毫针刺法】直刺 0.8 – 1.2 寸。

至阳

【标准定位】在脊柱区，第 7 胸椎棘突下凹陷中，后正中线上。

【毫针刺法】斜刺 0.5 ~ 1.0 寸，局部酸胀，可向下背或前胸放散。

4. Back

Combination Point　Dà Zhuī— Zhì Yáng.

Actions　Releasing the exterior and expelling wind.

DU 14 Dà Zhuī

Position　On the posterior midline of the neck, in the depression inferior to the spinous process of the seventh cervical vertebra.

Acupuncture　Insert the needle perpendicularly 0.8 ~ 1.2 cun deep.

DU 9 Zhì Yáng

Position　On the posterior midline of the back, in the depression inferior to the spinous process of the seventh thoracic vertebra.

Acupuncture　Insert the needle perpendicularly or obliquely 0.5 ~ 1.0 cun deep and stimulate until there is a sore and numbing sensation in the local area spreading to the back and chest.

第一章 内科病证
Chapter 1　Medical diseases

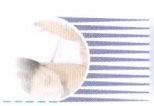

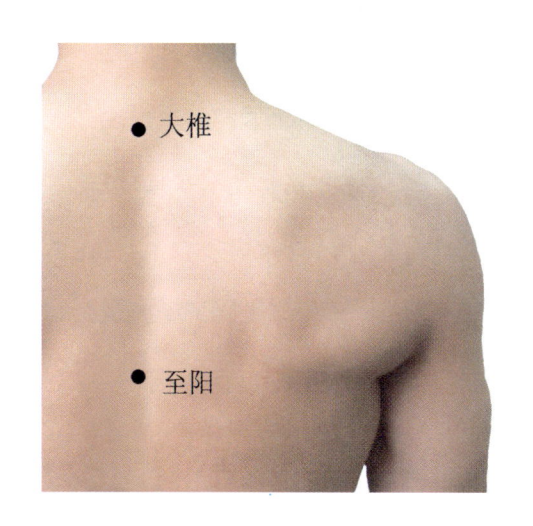

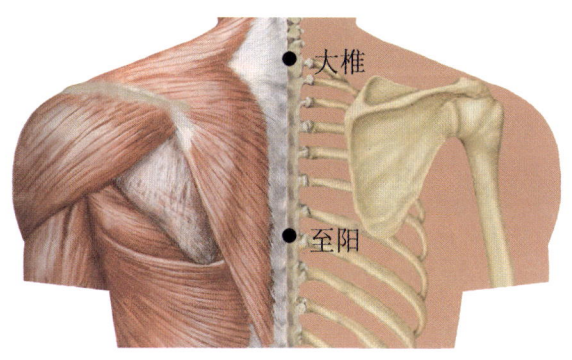

图 1-32-4　大椎—至阳

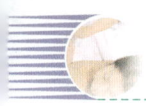

5. 髋部

组合穴　居髎—环跳。

功　能　强壮腰膝,通利关节。

居髎

【标准定位】髂前上棘与股骨大转子高点连线的中点。

【毫针刺法】直刺 1~1.5 寸。

环跳

【标准定位】在臀区,股骨大转子最凸点与骶管裂孔连线上的外 1/3 与 2/3 交点处。

【毫针刺法】直刺 2.0~3.0 寸,局部酸胀。

5. Hip

Combination Point　Jū Liáo—Huán Tiào.

Actions　Strenthening lumbar region, Activating the channel and benefiting joints.

GB 29 Jū Liáo

Position　On the hip, at the midpoint of the line connecting the anterior superior iliac spine and the great trochanter of the femur.

Acupuncture　Insert the needle perpendicularly 1~1.5 cun deep.

GB 30 Huán Tiào

Position　On the lateral aspect of the body when the thigh is flexed, at the junction of the lateral 1/3 and medial 2/3 of the line connecting the greater trochanter and the hiatus of the sacrum.

Acupuncture　Insert the needle obliquely downwards 2.0~3.0cun deep and stimulate until there is a sore and numbing sensation in the local area.

第一章 内科病证
Chapter 1 Medical diseases

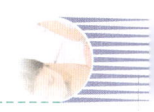

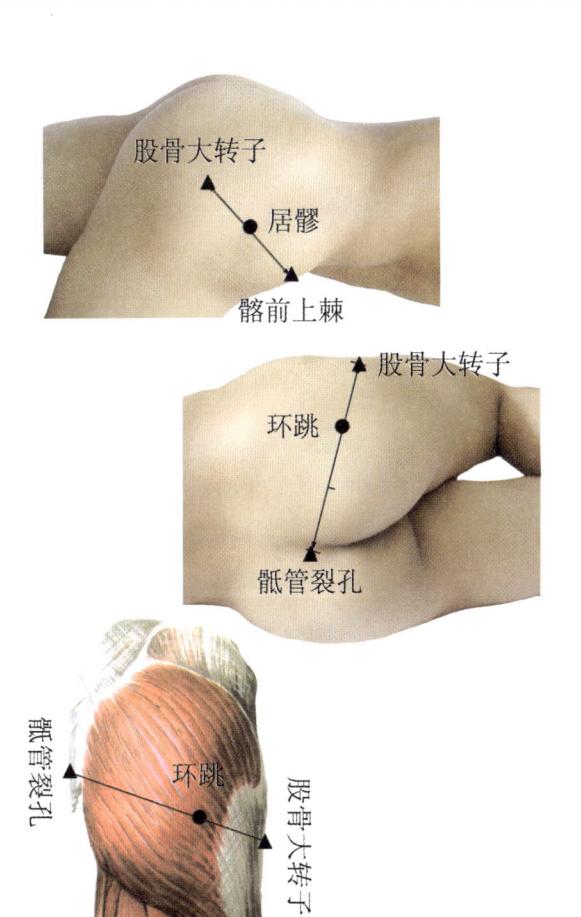

图 1-32-5 居髎—环跳

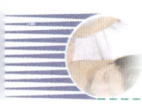

6. 股部

组合穴 环跳—承扶。

功　能 祛风除湿，强壮腰腿。

环跳

【标准定位】在臀区，股骨大转子最凸点与骶管裂孔连线上的外1/3与2/3交点处。

【毫针刺法】直刺2.0~3.0寸，局部酸胀。

承扶

【标准定位】在股后区，臀横纹的中点。

【毫针刺法】直刺1.5~2.5寸，局部酸胀。

6. Thigh

Combination Point　Huán Tiào— Chéng Fú.

Actions　Dispelling wind-dampness activates, Strenthening lumbar region.

GB 30 Huán Tiào

Position　On the lateral aspect of the body when the thigh is flexed, at the junction of the lateral 1/3 and medial 2/3 of the line connecting the greater trochanter and the hiatus of the sacrum.

Acupuncture　Insert the needle obliquely downwards 2.0~3.0 cun deep and stimulate until there is a sore and numbing sensation in the local area.

BL 36 Chéng Fú

Position　On the posterior side of the thigh, in the middle of the transverse gluteal fold.

Acupuncture　Insert the needle perpendicularly 1.5-2.5 cun deep and stimulate until there is a sore and numbing sensation in the local area radiating to the foot.

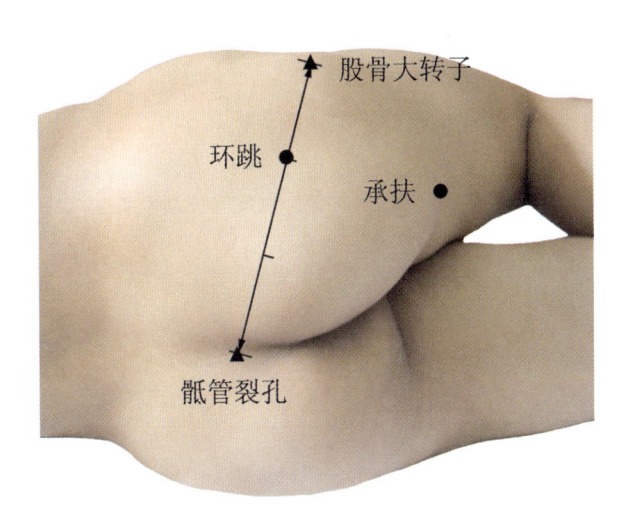

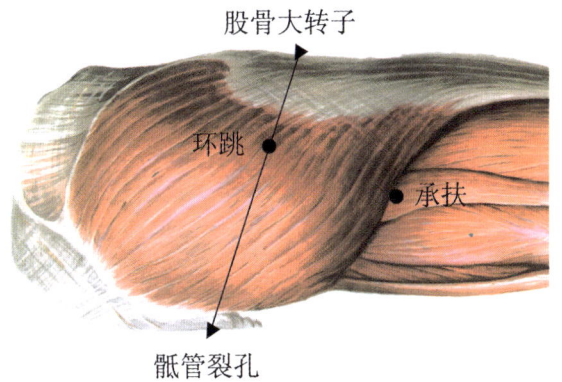

股骨大转子

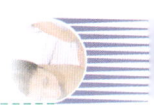

环跳

承扶

骶管裂孔

股骨大转子

环跳

承扶

骶管裂孔

图1-32-6 环跳—承扶

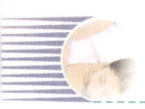

7. 膝部

组合穴 血海—梁丘。

功　能 活血化瘀，疏风止痛。

血海

【标准定位】屈膝，在大腿内侧，髌底内侧端上 2 寸，当股四头肌内侧头的隆起处。

【毫针刺法】直刺 1.0～2.0 寸，局部酸胀。

梁丘

【标准定位】在髂前上棘与髌骨底外缘连线上，当髌底上 2 寸处。

【毫针刺法】直刺 1.0～1.5 寸。

7. Knee

Combination Point　Xuè Hǎi— Liáng Qiū.

Actions　Promoting blood flow and dispelling stasis, expelling wind and alleviating pain.

SP 10 Xuè Hǎi

Position　In the medial aspect of the thigh, 2 cun proximal to the medial edge of the patella, on the bulge of the medial portion of m. quadriceps femoris when the knee is flexed.

Acupuncture　Insert the needle perpendicularly 1.0～2.0 cun deep.

ST 34 Liáng Qiū

Position　On the anterior aspect of the thigh, on the line connecting the anterior superior iliac spine and lateral end of the patella, 2 cun proximal to the patella when the knee is bent.

Acupuncture　Insert the needle perpendicularly 1.0～1.5 cun deep.

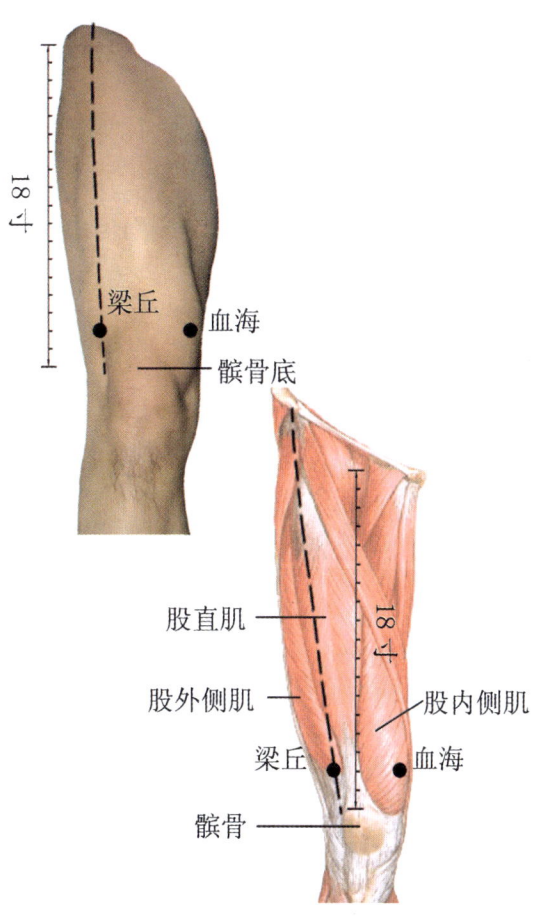

图 1-32-7 血海—梁丘

第三十三节 腰 痛

组合穴 委中—人中。

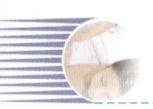

功 能 强壮腰膝,清热止痛。

委中

【标准定位】腘横纹中点,当股二头肌腱与半腱肌的中间。

【毫针刺法】直刺 0.5~1 寸。

人中(水沟)

【标准定位】在面部,人中沟的上 1/3 与中 1/3 交点处。

【毫针刺法】向上斜刺 0.2~0.3 寸,局部酸胀。

Section 33 Lumbago

Combination Point   Wěi Zhōng— Chéng Shān.

Actions   Benefiting the lumbar region and knees, Clearing heat and alleviating pain.

BL 40 Wěi Zhōng

Position   At the midpoint of the transverse crease of the popliteal fossa, between the tendon of m. biceps femoris and m. semitendinous.

Acupuncture   Insert the needle perpendicularly 0.5~1.0 cun deep.

DU 26 Shuǐ Gōu

Position   On the face, at the junction of the superior 1/3 and inferior 2/3 of the philtrum.

Acupuncture   Insert the needle obliquely upwards 0.2~0.3 cun deep and stimulate until there is a sore and numbing sensation in the local area.

图 1-33　委中—人中

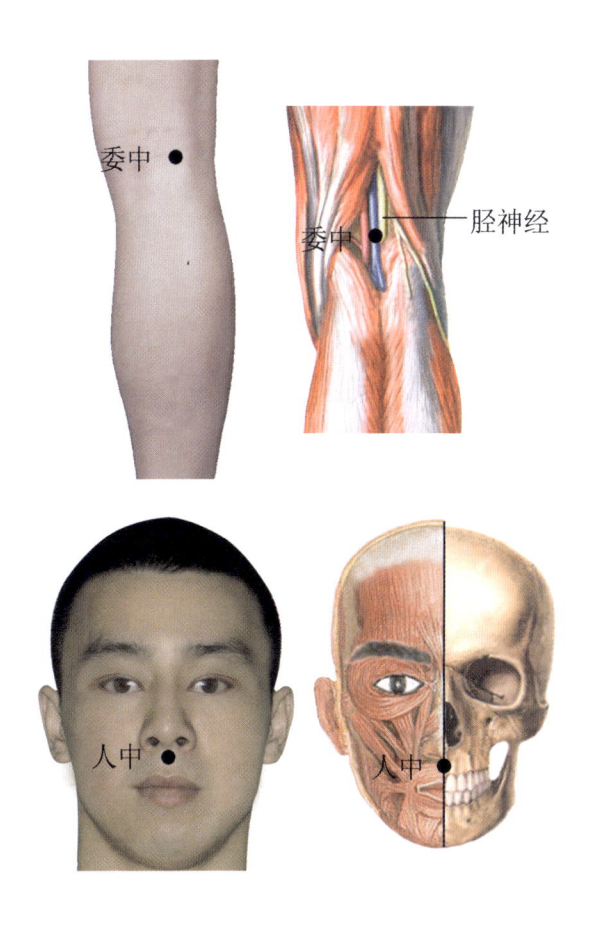

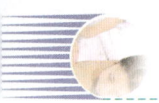

第三十四节 坐骨神经痛

组合穴 环跳—委中。
功 能 祛风除湿,强壮腰腿。

环跳
【标准定位】在臀区,股骨大转子最凸点与骶管裂孔连线上的外1/3与2/3交点处。
【毫针刺法】直刺2.0~3.0寸。

委中
【标准定位】腘横纹中点,当股二头肌腱与半腱肌的中间。
【毫针刺法】直刺0.5~1.0寸。

Section 34 Sciatica

Combination Point Huán Tiào— Chéng Fú.
Actions Dispelling wind – dampness, Strenthening lumbar region.

GB 30 Huán Tiào
Position On the lateral aspect of the body when the thigh is flexed, at the junction of the lateral 1/3 and medial 2/3 of the line connecting the greater trochanter and the hiatus of the sacrum.
Acupuncture Insert the needle obliquely downwards 1.0 ~ 3.0 cun deep.

BL 40 Wěi Zhōng
Position At the midpoint of the transverse crease of the popliteal fossa, between the tendon of m. biceps femoris and m. semitendinous.
Acupuncture Insert the needle perpendicularly 0.5 ~ 1.0 cun deep.

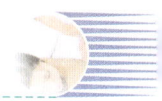

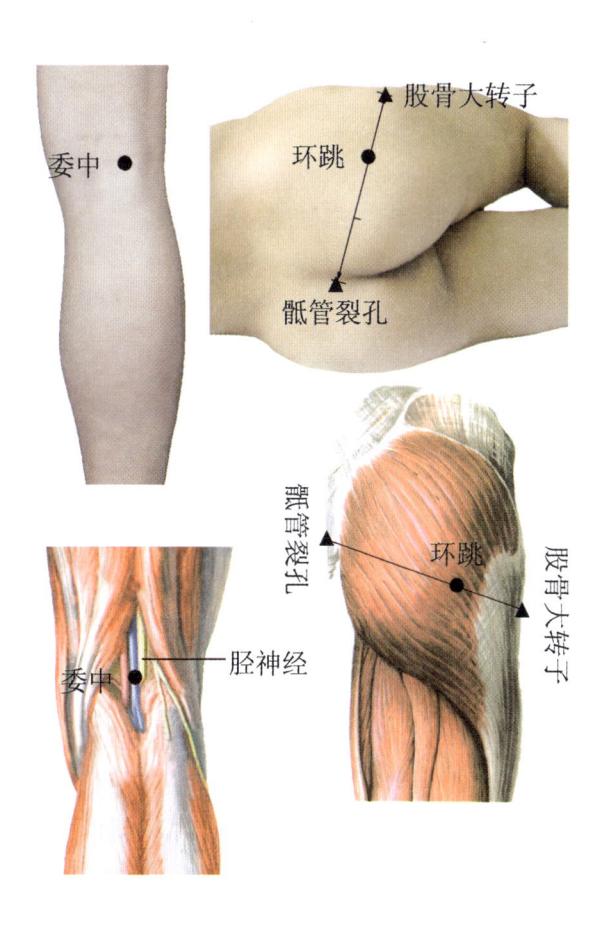

图 1-34 环跳—委中

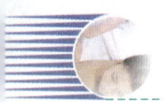

第三十五节 痿 证

1. 上肢

组合穴　曲池—合谷。

功　能　通利关节，祛风除湿。

曲池

【标准定位】在肘区，尺泽与肱骨外上髁上连线的中点处。

【毫针刺法】直刺1.0~2.0寸。

合谷

【标准定位】在手背，第2掌骨桡侧的中点处。

【毫针刺法】直刺0.5~1.0寸，局部酸胀。

Section 35　Flaccidity syndrome

1. The upper limbs

Combination Point　Qǔ Chí—Hé Gǔ.

Actions　Dispelling wind – dampness activating, the channel and benefiting the joint.

LI 11 Qǔ Chí

Position　In the depression of the radial side of the transverse cubital crease when elbow flexed.

Acupuncture　Insert the needle perpendicularly 1.0~2.0 cun deep.

LI 4 Hé Gǔ

Position　On the dorsum of the hand, between the first and second metacarpal bones, on the radial side of the middle of the second metacarpal bone.

Acupuncture　Insert the needle perpendicularly 0.5~1.0 cun deep.

第一章　内科病证
Chapter 1　Medical diseases

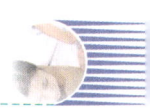

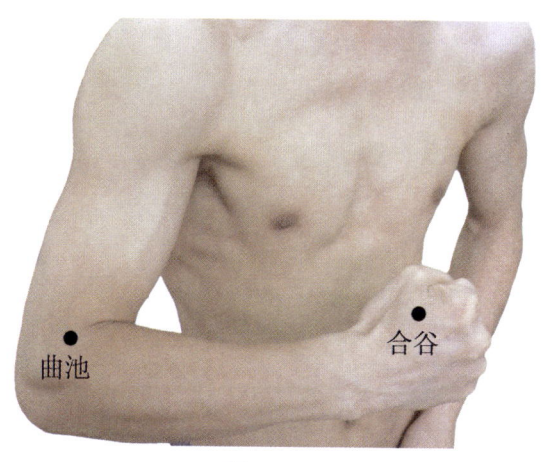

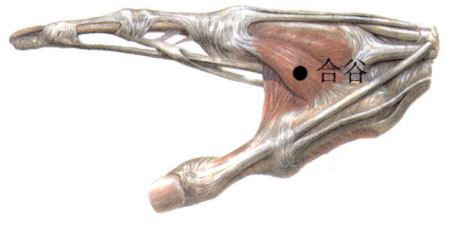

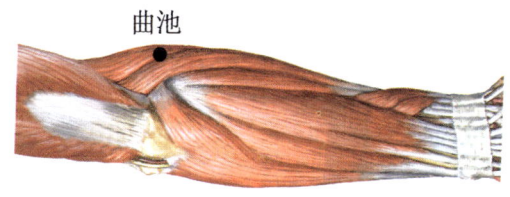

图 1-35-1　曲池—合谷

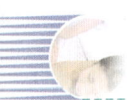

2. 下肢

组合穴 髀关—足三里。

功　能 舒筋通络，通利关节。

髀关

【标准定位】在股前区，股直肌近端、缝匠肌与阔筋膜张肌3条肌肉之间凹陷中。

【毫针刺法】直刺 1~1.5 寸。

足三里

【标准定位】在小腿外侧，犊鼻（ST 35）下 3 寸，犊鼻（ST 35）与解溪（ST 41）连线上。

【毫针刺法】直刺 0.5~1.5 寸，局部酸胀。

2. The lower limbs

Combination Point Bìguān—Zú Sān Lǐ.

Actions Activating the channel and benefiting joints.

ST 31 Bìguān

Position On the anterior aspect of the thigh, on the line connecting the anterior superior iliac spine and lateral end of the patella when the leg is flexed, in the notch lateral to the m. sartorius.

Acupuncture Insert the needle perpendicularly 1~1.5 cun deep.

ST36 Zú Sān Lǐ

Position On the anterior aspect of the lower leg, 3 cun distal to ST 35 (dú bí), one finger width lateral from the anterior ridge of the tibia.

Acupuncture Insert the needle perpendicularly 0.5~1.5 cun deep and stimulate until there is a sore and distending sensation.

第一章　内科病证
Chapter 1　Medical diseases

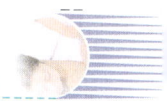

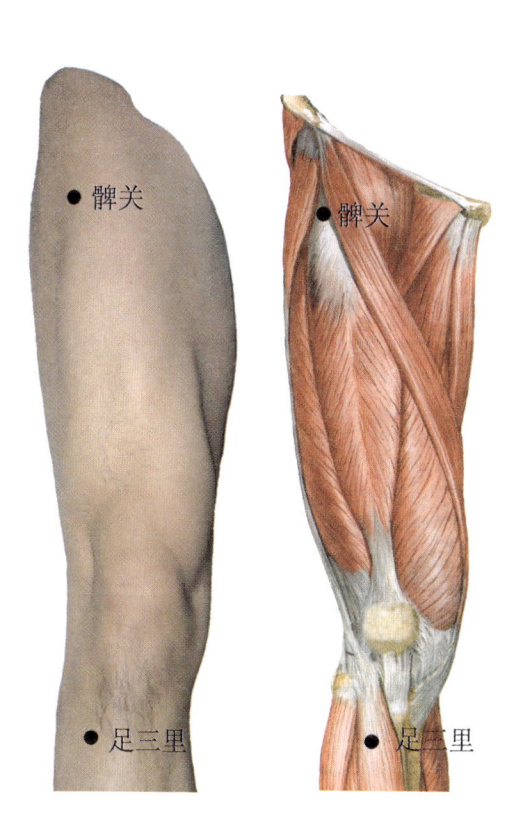

图 1-35-2　髀关—足三里

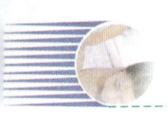

第三十六节 中 风

组合穴 人中—内关。

功 能 醒脑开窍,疏通气血。

人中(水沟)

【标准定位】在面部,人中沟的上 1/3 与中 1/3 交点处。

【毫针刺法】向上斜刺 0.2~0.3 寸,局部酸胀。

内关

【标准定位】在前臂前区,腕掌侧远端横纹上 2 寸,掌长肌腱与桡侧腕屈肌腱之间。

【毫针刺法】直刺 0.5~1.5 寸,局部酸胀。

Section 36 Apoplexy

Combination Point Shuǐ Gōu —Nèi Guān.

Actions activiting brain and regaining consciousness, Regulating qi and blood.

DU 26 Shuǐ Gōu

Position On the face, at the junction of the superior 1/3 and inferior 2/3 of the philtrum.

Acupuncture Insert the needle obliquely upwards 0.2 ~ 0.3 cun deep and stimulate until there is a sore and numbing sensation in the local area.

PC 6 Nèi Guān

Position On the palmar aspect of the forearm, 2 cun superior to the transverse crease of the wrist, between palmaris longus tendon and flexor carpi radialis tendon.

Acupuncture Insert the needle perpendicularly 0.5 ~ 1.5 cun deep and stimulate until there is a sore and numbing sensation.

第一章　内科病证
Chapter 1　Medical diseases

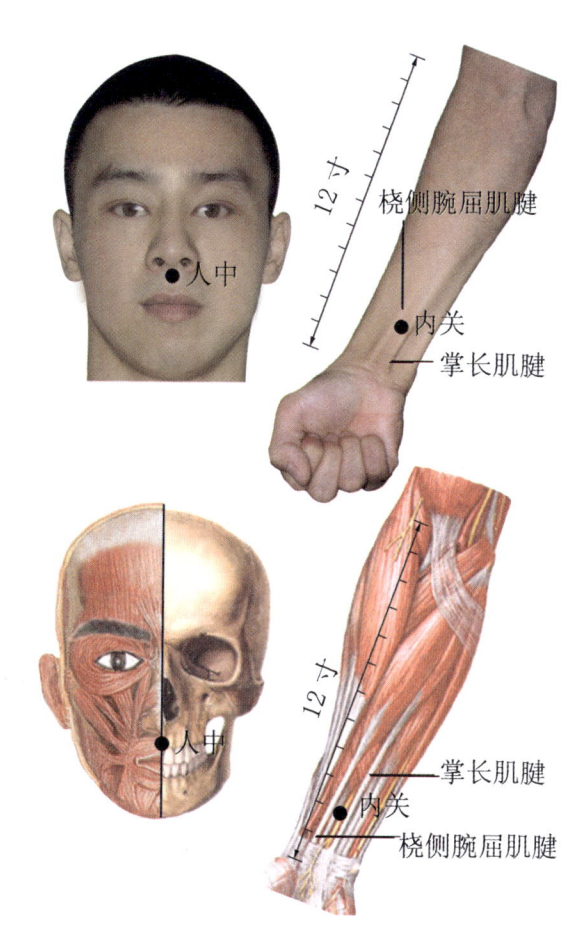

图 1-36　人中—内关

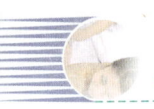

第三十七节 糖尿病

组合穴　胰俞—太溪。

功　能　清热润燥，益气养阴。

胰俞

【标准定位】在脊柱区，第8胸椎棘突下，后正中线旁开1.5寸。

【毫针刺法】斜刺0.5~1.0寸，局部酸胀。

太溪

【标准定位】在踝区，内踝尖与跟腱之间的凹陷中。

【毫针刺法】直刺0.3~0.5寸。

Section 37　Diabetes mellitus

Combination Point　Fēng Mén—Fèi Shū.

Actions　Clearing the heat and moistening dryness, benefiting the qi and nourishing yin.

Yíshú

Position　On the back, 1.5 cun lateral to the lower border of the spinous process of the eighth thoracic vertebra.

Acupuncture　Insert the needle obliquely towards the spine 0.5~1.0 cun deep.

KI 3 Tàixī

Position　On the medial aspect of the foot, posterior to the medial malleolus, in the depression between the tip of the medial malleolus and the tendon calcaneus.

Acupuncture　Insert the needle perpendicularly 0.3~0.5 cun deep.

图 1-37　胰俞—太溪

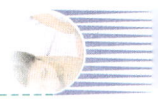

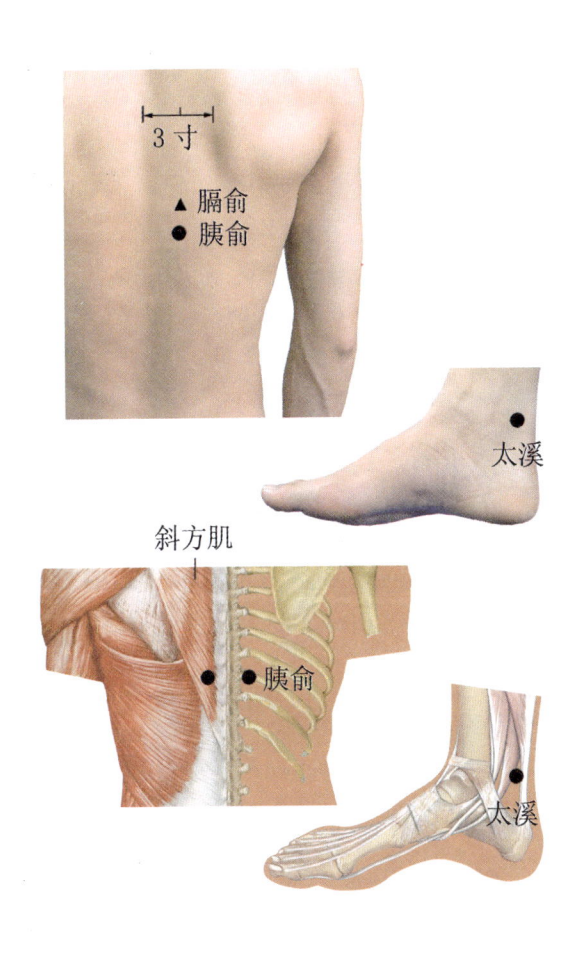

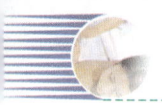

第三十八节 单纯性肥胖症

组合穴 中脘—天枢。
功 能 调中和胃。

中脘

【标准定位】在上腹部,脐中上4寸,前正中线上。
【毫针刺法】直刺0.5~1.0寸,局部酸胀沉重。

天枢

【标准定位】在腹部,横平脐中,前正中线旁开2寸。
【毫针刺法】直刺1.0~1.5寸,局部酸胀,可扩散至同侧腹部。

Section 38 Simple obesity

Combination Point Zhōng Wǎn —Tiān Shū.

Actions Harmonizing stomach and regulating qi.

RN12 Zhōng Wǎn

Position On the upper abdomen, on the anterior midline, 4 cun superior to the umbilicus.

Acupuncture Insert the needle perpendicularly 0.5 ~ 1.0 cun deep and stimulate until there is a sore and distending sensation in the local area.

ST 25 Tiān Shū

Position On the abdomen, 2 cun lateral to the umbilicus.

Acupuncture Insert the needle perpendicularly 1.0 ~ 1.5 cun deep and stimulate until there is a sore and numbing sensation in the local area radiating to the side of the abdomen.

图1-38 中脘—天枢

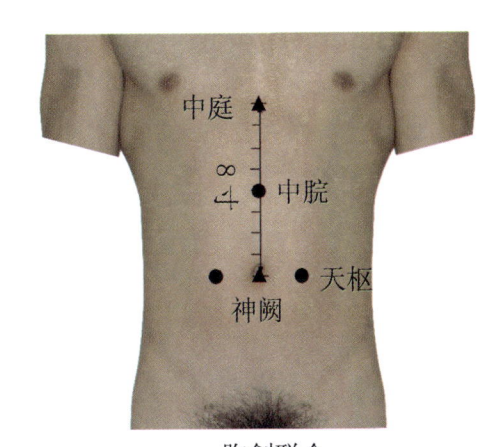

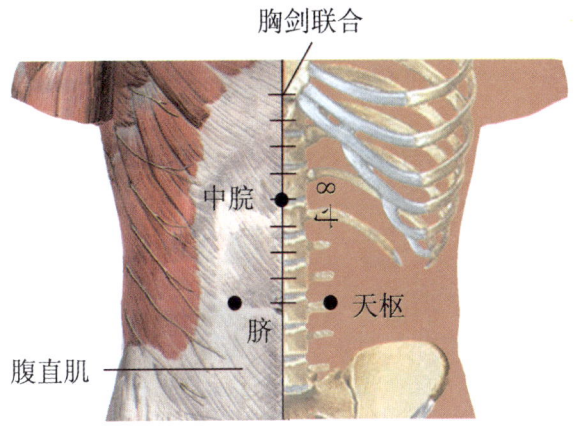

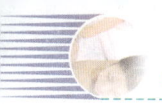

第二章 外科病证
Chapter 2　Surgical diseases

第一节　疔疮

组合穴　身柱—灵台。
功　能　解毒疗疮。

灵台
【标准定位】第 6 胸椎棘突下凹陷中，后正中线上。
【毫针刺法】斜刺 0.5～1.0 寸。

身柱
【标准定位】在脊柱区，第 3 胸椎棘突下凹陷中，后正中线上。
【毫针刺法】斜刺 0.5～1.0 寸。

Section 1　Malignant furuncle

Combination Point　Shēn Zhù—Líng Tái.

Actions　Detoxification and curing furuncles.

DU 12 Shēn Zhù

Position　On the posterior midline of the back, in the depression inferior to the spinous process of the third thoracic vertebra.

Acupuncture　Insert the needle obliquely 0.5～1.0 cun deep.

DU 10 Líng Tái.

Position　On the posterior midline of the back, in the depression inferior to the spinous process of the sixth thoracic vertebra.

Acupuncture　Insert the needle obliquely 0.5～1.0 cun deep.

图2-1 身柱—灵台

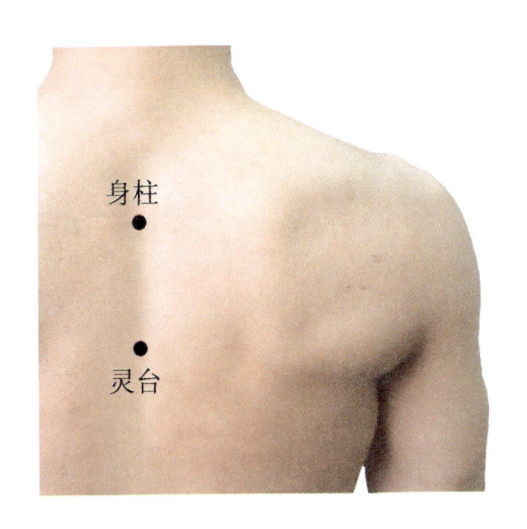

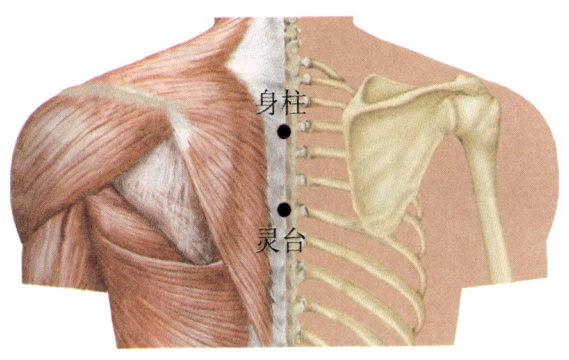

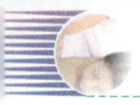

第二节 丹　毒

组合穴　合谷—曲池。

功　能　清热解毒。

合谷

【标准定位】在手背，第2掌骨桡侧的中点处。

【毫针刺法】直刺0.5～1.0寸，局部酸胀。

曲池

【标准定位】尺泽与肱骨外上髁上连线的中点处。

【毫针刺法】直刺1.0～2.0寸。

Section 2　Erysipelas

Combination Point　Hé Gǔ—Qǔ Chí.

Actions　clearing heat and removing toxicity.

LI 4 Hé Gǔ

Position　On the dorsum of the hand, between the first and second metacarpal bones, on the radial side of the middle of the second metacarpal bone.

Acupuncture　Insert the needle perpendicularly 0.5～1.0 cun deep.

LI 11 Qǔ Chí

Position　In the depression of the radial side of the transverse cubital crease when elbow flexed.

Acupuncture　Insert the needle perpendicularly 1.0～2.0 cun deep.

第二章 外科病证
Chapter 2　Surgical diseases

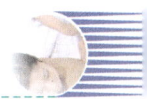

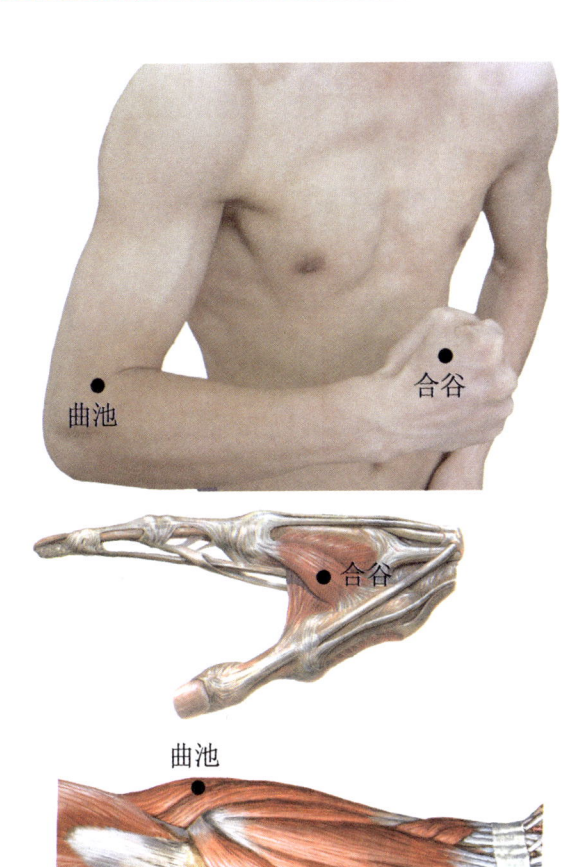

图 2-2　合谷—曲池

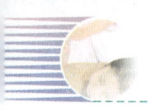

第三节　流行性腮腺炎

组合穴　合谷—翳风。

功　能　清热解毒，消肿散结。

合谷

【标准定位】在手背，第1、2掌骨间，第2掌骨桡侧的中点处。

【毫针刺法】直刺0.5～1.0寸。

翳风

【标准定位】耳垂后方，乳突下端前方凹陷中。

【毫针刺法】直刺0.8～1.2寸，耳后酸胀。

Section 3　Epidemic parotitis

Combination Point　Hé Gǔ— Yì Fēng.

Actions　clearing heat and removing toxicity, reducing swelling.

LI 4 Hé Gǔ

Position　On the dorsum of the hand, between the first and second metacarpal bones, on the radial side of the middle of the second metacarpal bone.

Acupuncture　Insert the needle perpendicularly 0.5～1.0 cun deep.

SJ 17 Yì Fēng

Position　Posterior to the lobule of the ear, in the depression between the mastoid process and the angle of the mandible.

Acupuncture　Insert the needle perpendicularly 0.8～1.2 cun deep and stimulate until there is a sore and numbing sensation in the local area.

第二章 外科病证
Chapter 2 Surgical diseases

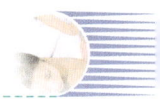

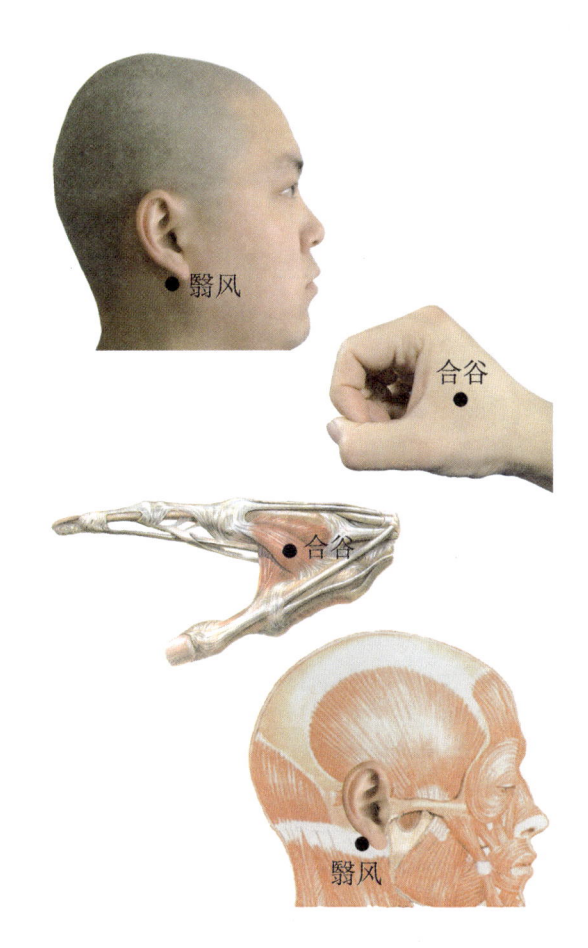

图 2-3 合谷—翳风

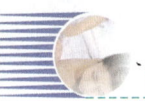

第四节　乳腺炎

组合穴　肩井—少泽。
功　能　清热解毒，消肿止痛。

肩井

【标准定位】在肩胛区，第 7 颈椎棘突与肩峰最外侧点连线的中点。

【毫针刺法】直刺或向四周斜刺 0.5～0.8 寸。

少泽

【标准定位】在手指，小指末节尺侧，距指甲根角侧上方 0.1 寸（指寸）。

【毫针刺法】直刺 0.1～0.2 寸。

Section 4　Mastitis

Combination Point　Jiānjǐng—Shàozé.

Actions　clearing heat, reducing swelling and alleviating pain.

GB 21 Jiānjǐng

Position　On the shoulder, at the midpoint of the line connecting DU 14 (dà zhuī) and the acromion end of the clavicle.

Acupuncture　Insert the needle subcutaneously 0.5～0.8 cun deep.

SI 1 Shàozé

Position　On the ulnar side of the distal phalanx of the little finger, 0.1 cun lateral to the corner of the nail.

Acupuncture　Insert the needle 0.1～0.2 cun deep.

第二章 外科病证
Chapter 2 Surgical diseases

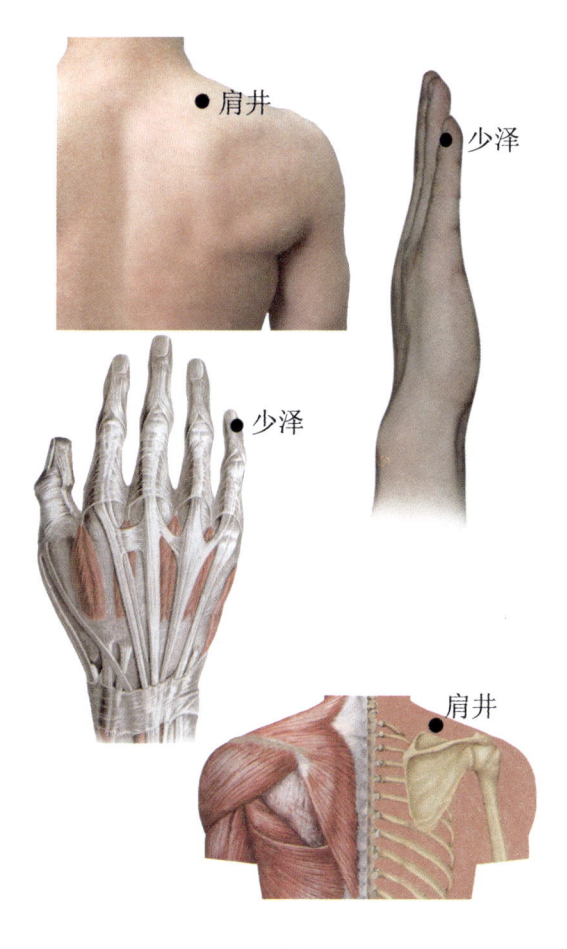

图 2-4 肩井—少泽

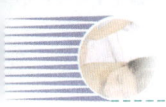

第五节　乳腺增生病

组合穴　期门—膻中。

功　能　疏肝解郁，理气降逆。

期门

【标准定位】第 6 肋间隙，前正中线旁开 4 寸。

【毫针刺法】斜刺 0.5～0.8 寸。

膻中

【标准定位】在胸部，当前正中线上，平第四肋间，两乳头连线的中点。

【毫针刺法】平刺 0.3～0.5 寸。

Section 5　Hyperplastic disease of breast

Combination Point　Qī Mén—Tán Zhōng.

Actions　Spreading liver and regulating qi.

LV14 Qī Mén

Position　On the chest, directly inferior to the nipple, in the sixth intercostal space, 4 cun lateral to the anterior midline.

Acupuncture　Insert the needle obliquely or along the intercostals space 0.5～0.8 cun.

RN17 Tán Zhōng

Position　On the chest, on the anterior midline, at the level of the fourth intercostal space, at the midpoint between the two nipples.

Acupuncture　Insert the needle subcutaneously or obliquely 0.3～0.5 cun deep.

第二章 外科病证
Chapter 2 Surgical diseases

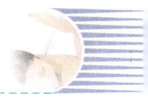

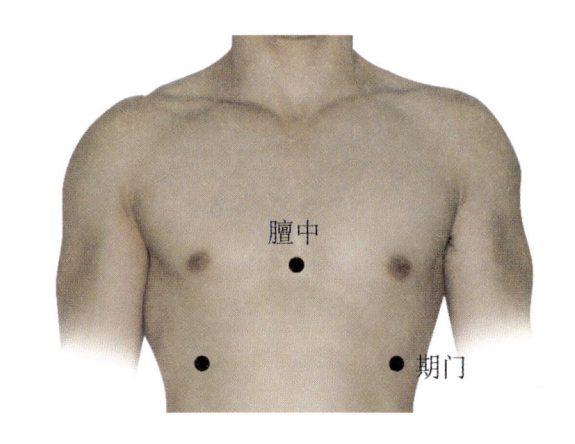

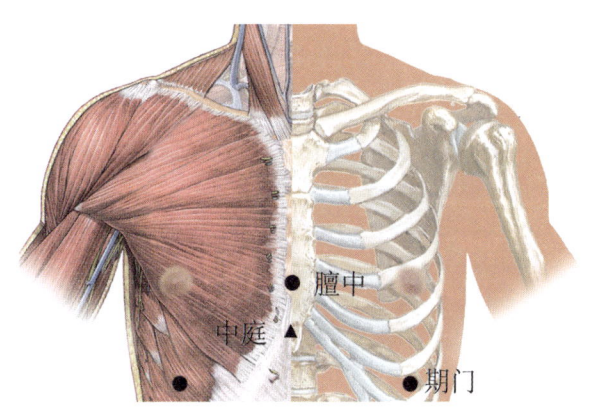

图 2-5 期门—膻中

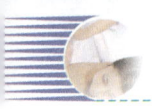

第六节 胆石症

组合穴 阳陵泉—胆囊穴。

功　能 疏肝利胆，行气止痛。

阳陵泉

【标准定位】在小腿外侧，腓骨头前下方凹陷中。

【毫针刺法】向内斜刺 0.5~0.8 寸，局部酸胀。

胆囊穴

【标准定位】在小腿外侧，阳陵泉穴直下 2 寸。

【毫针刺法】直刺 1.0~1.5 寸，局部酸胀。

Section 6　Cholelithiasis

Combination Point　Yáng líng quán—Dǎn náng xuè.

Actions　Spreading liver and Clearing gall bladder heat.

GB 34　Yánglíngquán

Position　On the anterior aspect of the lower leg, in the depression anterior and inferior to the head of the fibula.

Acupuncture　Insert the needle obliquely 0.5 ~ 0.8 cun deep and stimulate until there is a sore and numbing sensation in the local area.

EX – LE 8　Dǎnnángxuè

Position　In the depression approximately 2 cun inferior to GB 34 (yang ling quán).

Acupuncture　Insert the needle perpendicularly 1.0 – 1.5 cun deep and stimulate until there is a sore and heavy sensation in the local area.

第二章 外科病证
Chapter 2 Surgical diseases

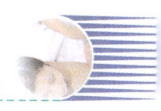

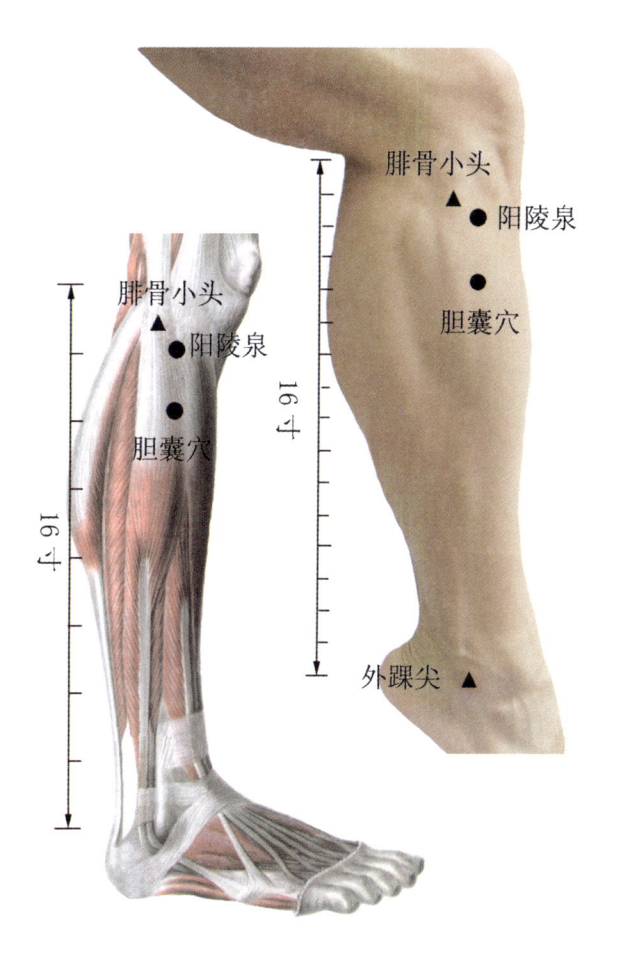

图 2-6 阳陵泉—胆囊穴

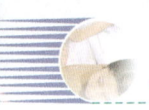

第七节 阑尾炎

组合穴 天枢—阑尾穴。
功 能 理气通腑止痛。

天枢
【标准定位】在腹部,横平脐中,前正中线旁开2寸。
【毫针刺法】直刺1.0~1.5寸,局部酸胀,可扩散至同侧腹部。

阑尾穴
【标准定位】在小腿外侧,足三里下5寸。
【毫针刺法】直刺0.5~1.0寸,局部酸胀。

Section 7　Appendicitis

Combination Point　Tiān Shū—Lán wěi xuè.

Actions　regulating qi and fu – organs, alleviating pain.

ST 25 Tiān Shū

Position　On the abdomen, 2 cun lateral to the umbilicus.

Acupuncture　Insert the neelde perpendicularly 1.0 ~ 1.5 cun deep and stimulate until there is a sore and numbing sensation in the local area radiating to the side of the abdomen.

EX – LE7 Lán wěi xuè

Position　The tender depression approximately 2 cun distal to ST 36 (zú sān lǐ).

Acupuncture　Insert the needle perpendicularly 0.5 – 1.0 cun deep and stimulate until there is a sore and heavy sensation in the local area.

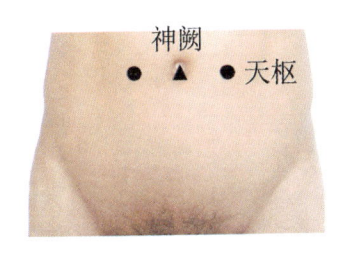

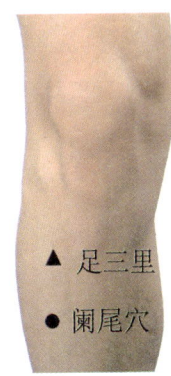

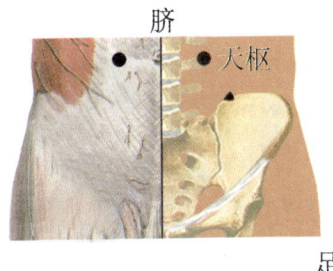

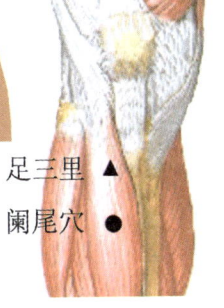

图 2-7 天枢—阑尾

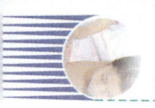

第八节　疝　气

组合穴　大敦—太冲。
功　能　理气除疝。

大敦

【标准定位】在足趾,大趾末节外侧,趾甲根角侧后方0.1寸(指寸)。

【毫针刺法】直刺0.1~0.2寸。

太冲

【标准定位】在足背,当第1、2跖骨间,跖骨底结合部前方凹陷中。

【毫针刺法】向上斜刺0.5~1.0,局部酸胀。

Section 8　Hernia

Combination Point　Dàdūn —Tài Chōng.

Actions　Regulating qi and dispelling hernia.

LV 1 Dàdūn

Position　On the foot, 0.1 cun lateral to the corner of the nail of the big toe.

Acupuncture　Insert the needle subcutaneously 0.1~0.2 cun deep.

LV 3 Tài Chōng

Position　On the dorsum of the foot, in the depression proximal to the first metatarsal space.

Acupuncture　Insert the needle obliquely upwards 0.5~1.0 cun deep and stimulate until there is a sore and numbing sensation.

第二章　外科病证
Chapter 2　Surgical diseases

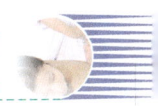

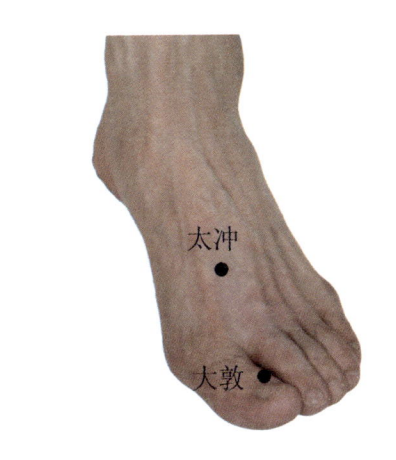

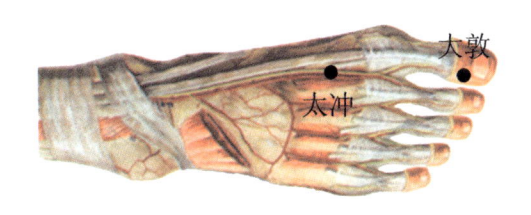

图 2-8　大敦—太冲

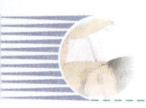

第九节 痔 疮

组合穴 大肠俞—秩边。
功 能 清热化痔。

大肠俞
【标准定位】第4腰椎棘突下,后正中线旁开1.5寸。
【毫针刺法】直刺0.8~1.0寸,局部酸胀。

秩边
【标准定位】横平第4骶后孔,骶正中嵴旁开3寸。
【毫针刺法】直刺1.5~3.0寸,局部酸胀。

Section 9　Haemorrhoids

Combination Point　Dà Cháng Shū— Zhì Biān.

Actions　Clearing the heat and treating hemorrhoids.

BL 25 Dà Cháng Shū

Position　On the lower back, 1.5 cun lateral to the lower border of the spinous process of the fourth lumbar vertebra.

Acupuncture　Insert the needle perpendicularly 0.8 ~ 1.0 cun deep.

BL 54 Zhì Biān

Position　On the lower back, 3 cun lateral to the middle sacral creast, at the level with the fourth posterior sacral foramen.

Acupuncture　Insert the needle perpendicularly obliquely 1.5 ~ 3.0 cun deep and stimulate until there is a sore and numbing sensation in the local area.

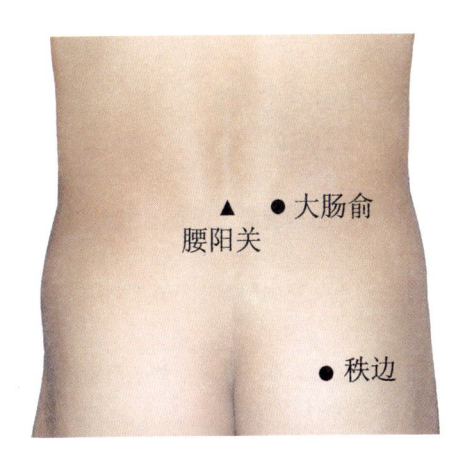

大肠俞
腰阳关

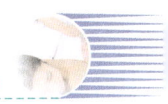

秩边

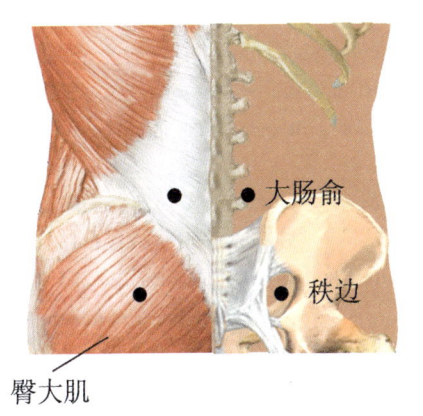

臀大肌　　大肠俞

秩边

图 2-9　大肠俞—秩边

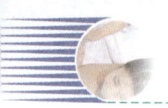

第十节 脱 肛

组合穴 百会—承山。

功 能 益气升提固脱。

百会

【标准定位】在头部,当前发际正中直上5寸,或两耳尖连线的中点处。

【毫针刺法】平刺,针尖可向四周进针0.5~0.8寸。

承山

【标准定位】在小腿后区,腓肠肌两肌腹与肌腱交角处。

【毫针刺法】直刺1.0~1.5寸。

Section 10 Prolapse of anus

Combination Point Bǎi Huì—Chéngshān.

Actions Calming the spirit and countering prolapse.

DU 20 Bǎi Huì

Position On the head, 5 cun posterior to the midpoint of the anterior hairline, and at the midpoint of the line between the two ears.

Acupuncture Insert the needle subcutaneously 0.5~0.8 cun deep and stimulate until there is a sore and distending sensation in the local area.

BL 57 Chéngshān

Position On the posterior midline of the lower leg, in the depression of the belly of the m. gastrocnemius when the toes are extended or the heel is lifted from the ground.

Acupuncture Insert the needle obliquely 1.0~1.5 cun deep.

图 2-10 百会—承山

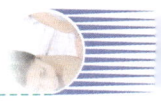

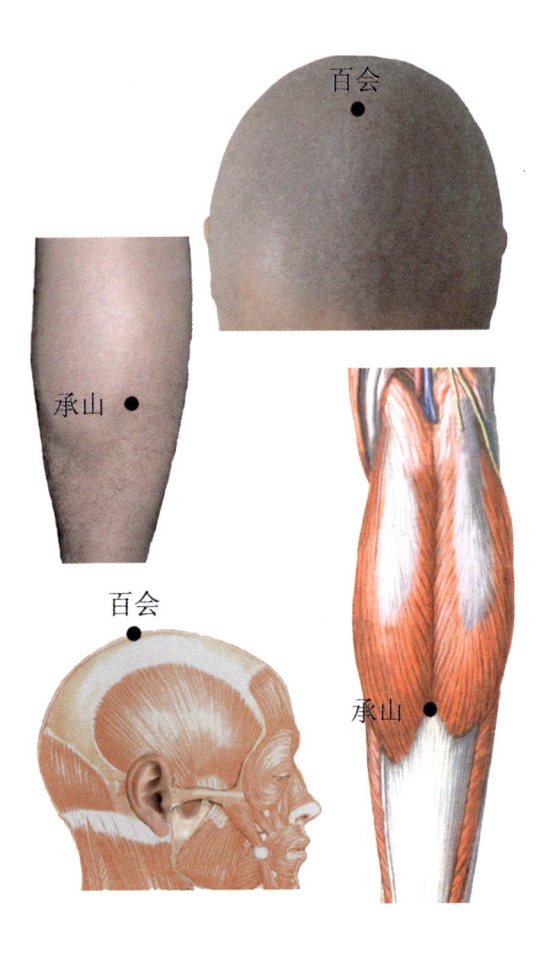

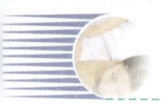

第三章 妇科、男科病证
Chapter 3　Gynecological and male diseases

第一节　月经不调

组合穴　足三里—三阴交。
功　能　补气活血调经。

足三里
【标准定位】犊鼻下3寸，犊鼻与解溪连线上。
【毫针刺法】直刺0.5～1.5寸，局部酸胀。

三阴交
【标准定位】在小腿内侧，当足内踝尖上3寸。
【毫针刺法】直刺1.0～1.5寸。

Section 1　Irregular menstruation

Combination Point　Zú Sān Lǐ— Sān Yīn Jiāo.

Actions　Tonifying qi , Promoting blood flow, restoring menstrual flow.

ST 36 Zú Sān Lǐ

Position　On the anterior aspect of the lower leg, 3 cun distal to ST 35 (dú bí), one finger width lateral from the anterior ridge of the tibia.

Acupuncture　Insert the needle perpendicularly 0.5～1.5 cun deep.

Chapter 3 Gynecological and male diseases

SP 6 Sān Yīn Jiāo

Position　On the medial part of the leg, 3 cun superior to the tip of medial malleolus, posterior to the medial edge of the tibia.

Acupuncture　Insert the needle perpendicularly 0.5~1.0 cun deep.

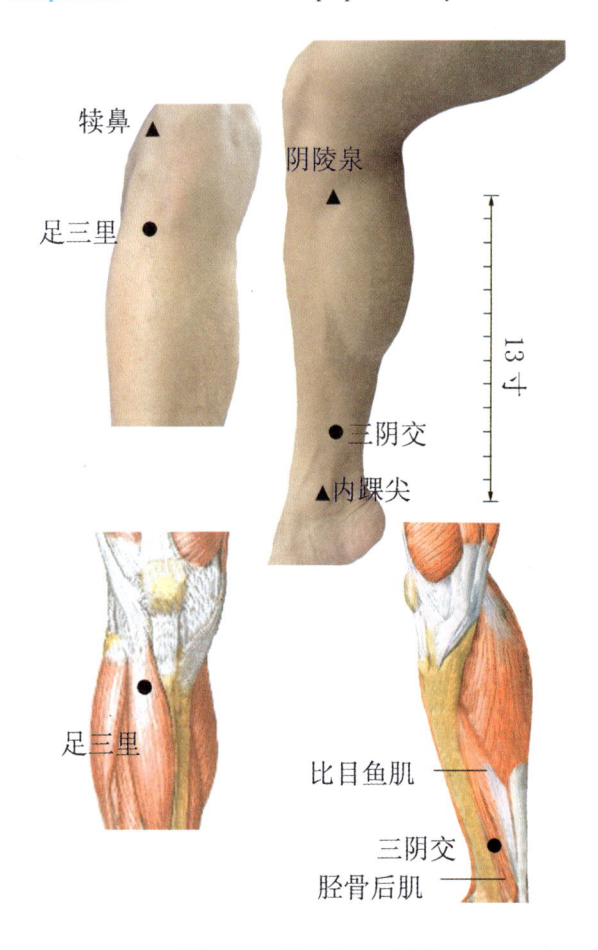

图 3-1　足三里—三阴交

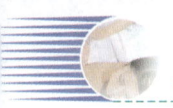

第二节 痛 经

组合穴 十七椎—三阴交。

功 能 行气活血止痛。

十七椎

【标准定位】 在腰区,当后正中线上,第 5 腰椎棘突下凹陷中。

【毫针刺法】 直刺 0.8～1.2 寸,局部酸胀。

三阴交

【标准定位】 当足内踝尖上 3 寸,胫骨内侧缘后方。

【毫针刺法】 直刺 1.0～1.5 寸。孕妇不宜针。

Section 2　Dysmenorrhea

Combination Point　Shíqīzhuī—Sān Yīn Jiāo.

Actions　regulating qi, promotes blood flow and alleviating pain.

EX – B 12 Shíqīzhuī

Position　On the back, along the posterior midline, inferior to the spinous process of the fifth lumbar vertebra.

Acupuncture　Insert the needle perpendicularly 0.8 – 1.2 cun deep and stimulate until there is a sore and heavy sensation in the local area.

SP 6 Sān Yīn Jiāo

Position　On the medial part of the leg, 3 cun superior to the tip of medial malleolus, posterior to the medial edge of the tibia.

Acupuncture　Insert the needle perpendicularly 0.5～1.5 cun deep and stimulate until there is a sore and numbing sensation in the local area.

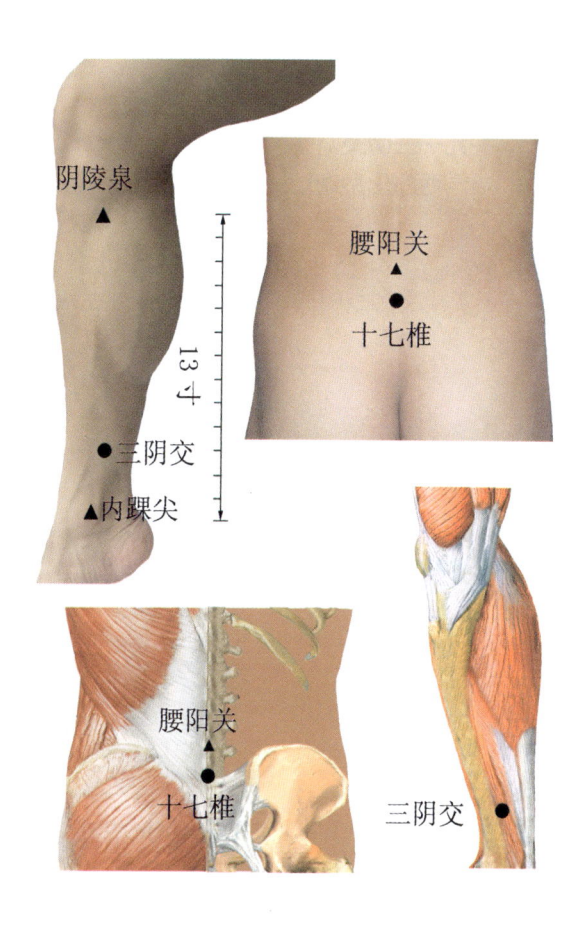

图3-2 十七椎—三阴交

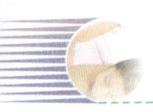

第三节 闭 经

组合穴 关元—三阴交。
功 能 益气活血化瘀调经。

关元
【标准定位】在下腹部,脐中下3寸,前正中线上。
【毫针刺法】需排尿后进行针刺。直刺0.5~1.0寸,局部酸胀,可放射至外生殖器和会阴部。

三阴交
【标准定位】当足内踝尖上3寸,胫骨内侧缘后方。
【毫针刺法】直刺1.0~1.5寸。孕妇不宜针。

Section 3 Amenorrhoea

Combination Point Guān Yuán—Sān Yīn Jiāo.

Actions benefiting qi and Promoting blood flow and dispelling stasis, regulating menstruation.

RN4 Guān Yuán

Position On the lower abdomen, on the anterior midline, 3 cun inferior to the umbilicus.

Acupuncture Insert the needle after the micturition, perpendicularly 0.5~1.0 cun deep and stimulate until there is a sore and distending sensation in the local area radiating to the genitalia.

SP 6 Sān Yīn Jiāo

Position On the medial part of the leg, 3 cun superior to the tip of medial malleolus, posterior to the medial edge of the tibia.

Acupuncture Insert the needle perpendicularly 0.5~1.5 cun deep and stimulate until there is a sore and numbing sensation in the local area.

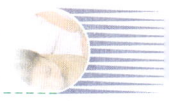

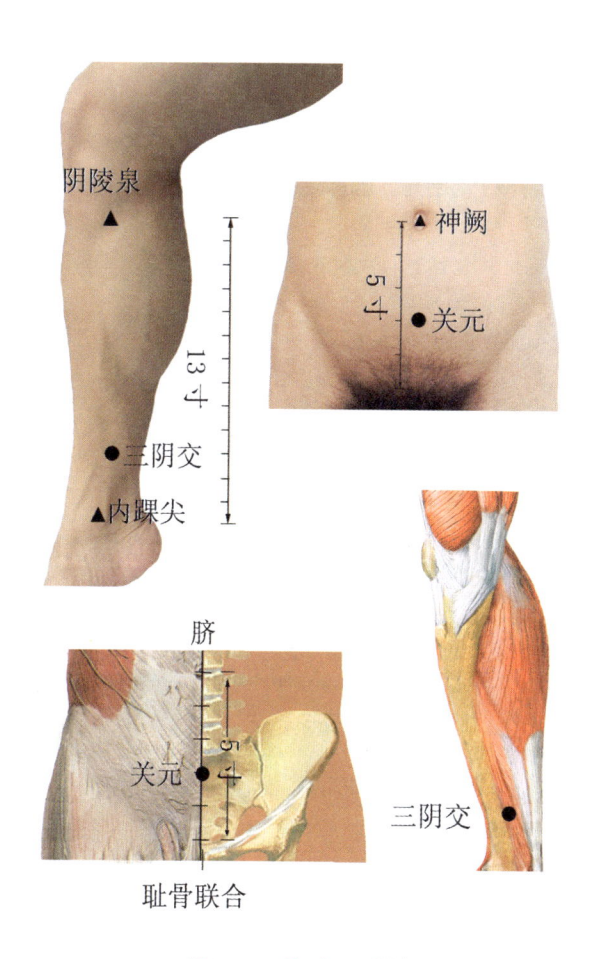

第三章　妇科、男科病证
Chapter 3　Gynecological and male diseases

图 3-3　关元—三阴交

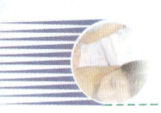

第四节 崩 漏

组合穴 隐白—关元。

功 能 补气培元,固冲止血。

隐白

【标准定位】在足趾,大趾末节内侧,趾甲根角侧后方0.1寸(指寸)。

【毫针刺法】直刺0.1~0.2寸。

关元

【标准定位】在下腹部,脐中下3寸,前正中线上。

【毫针刺法】需排尿后进行针刺。直刺0.5~1.0寸,局部酸胀,可放射至外生殖器和会阴部。

Section 4　Metrorrhagia

Combination Point　Yǐnbái— Guān Yuán.

Actions　Tonifying original qi and benefiting essence, invigorating the chong meridian to cure metrorrhagia.

SP 1 Yǐnbái

Position　On the medial side of the the big toe, 0.1 cun lateral to the corner of the nail.

Acupuncture　Insert the needle 0.1~0.2 cun deep.

RN 4 Guān Yuán

Position　On the lower abdomen, on the anterior midline, 3 cun inferior to the umbilicus.

Acupuncture　Insert the needle perpendicularly 0.5~1.0 cun deep and stimulate until there is a sore and distending sensation in the local area radiating to the genitalia.

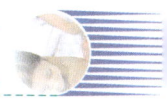

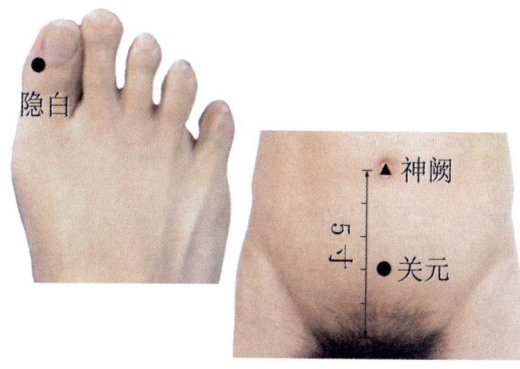

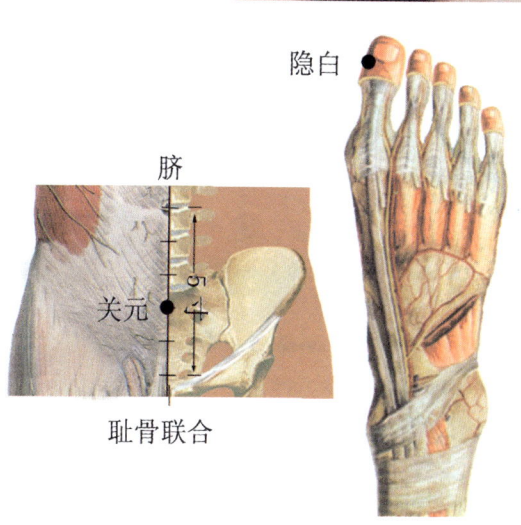

第三章 妇科、男科病证
Chapter 3 Gynecological and male diseases

图 3-4 隐白—关元

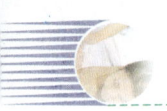

第五节　带下病

组合穴　中极—带脉。
功　能　渗湿止带。

中极

【标准定位】在下腹部，脐中下 4 寸，前正中线上。

【毫针刺法】直刺 0.5～1.0 寸，局部酸胀，可放射至外生殖器和会阴部。

带脉

【标准定位】在侧腹部，第 11 肋骨游离端垂线与脐水平线的交点上。

【毫针刺法】直刺 0.5～1.0 寸。

Section 5　Leucorrhoea disease

Combination Point　Zhōng Jí—Dài Mài.

Actions　Transforming dampness and regulating the leucorrhoea.

RN 3 Zhōng Jí.

Position　On the lower abdomen, on the anterior midline, 4 cun inferior to the umbilicus.

Acupuncture　Insert the needle perpendicularly 0.5～1.0 cun deep and stimulate until there is a sore and distending sensation in the local area radiating to the genitalia.

GB 26 Dàimài

Position　Below the free end of the eleventh floating rib, at the level with the umbilicus.

Acupuncture　Insert the needle obliquely 0.5～1.0 cun deep.

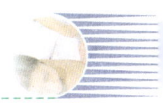

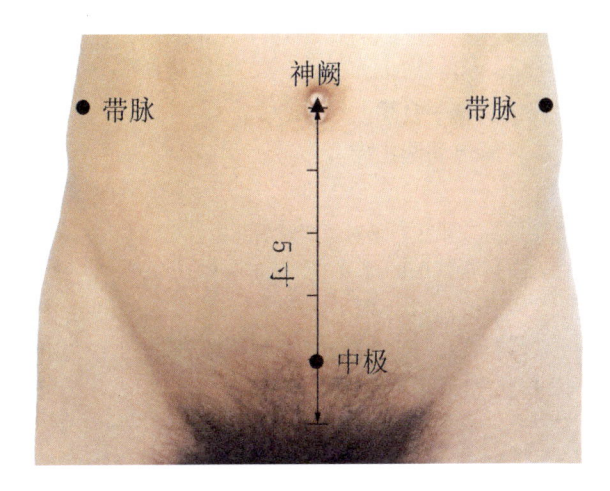

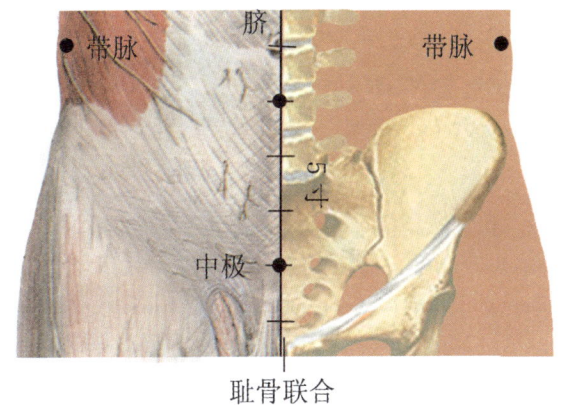

第三章 妇科、男科病证
Chapter 3　Gynecological and male diseases

图 3-5　中极—带脉

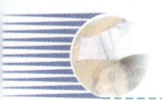

第六节 阴 痒

组合穴 次髎—会阴。
功 能 清热利湿止痒。

次髎
【标准定位】 在骶区,正对第2骶后孔中。
【毫针刺法】 直刺0.8~1.0寸,骶部酸胀。

会阴
【标准定位】 在会阴区。男性在阴囊根部与肛门连线的中点,女性在大阴唇后联合与肛门连线的中点。
【毫针刺法】 直刺0.8~1.0寸,局部酸胀。

Section 6　Pruritus vulvae

Combination Point 　Cì Liáo—Huì Yīn.

Actions 　Clearing heat and removing damp, relieving itching.

BL 32 Cì Liáo

Position 　On the sacrum, medial and superior to the superior iliac spine, in the depression of the second posterior sacral foramen.

Acupuncture 　Insert the needle perpendicularly 0.5~0.8 cun deep and stimulate until there is a sore and numbing sensation in the local area.

RN 1 Huì Yīn

Position 　On the perineum, at the midpoint between the anus and the root of the scrotum in males and between the anus and the posterior labial commissure in females.

Acupuncture 　Insert the needle perpendicularly 0.5~1.0 cun deep.

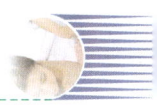

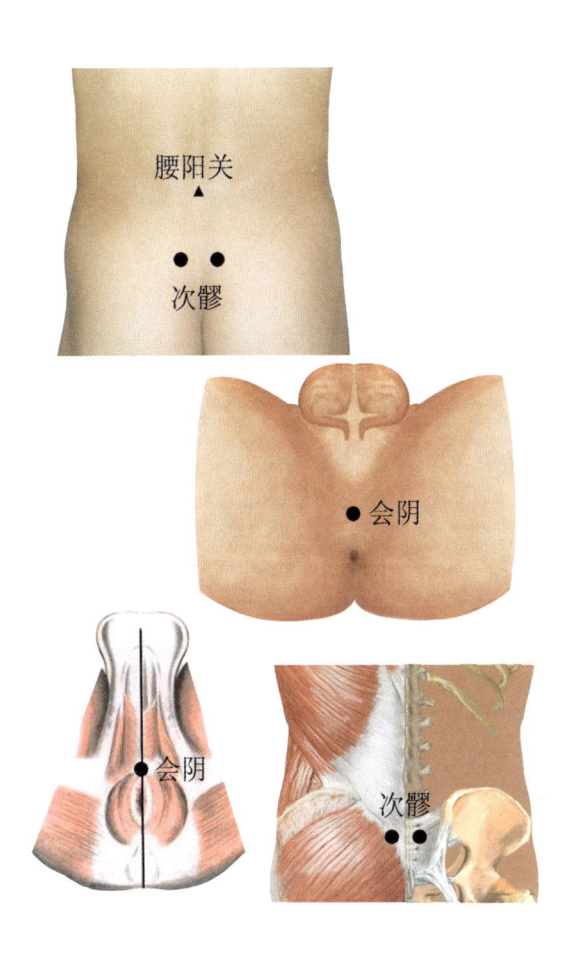

第三章 妇科、男科病证
Chapter 3　Gynecological and male diseases

图 3-6　次髎—会阴

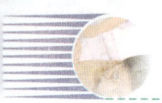

第七节 子宫脱垂

组合穴 百会—子宫。

功 能 明目益智,开窍宁神。

百会

【标准定位】在头部,当前发际正中直上5寸,或两耳尖连线的中点处。

【毫针刺法】平刺,针尖可向四周进针0.5~0.8寸。

子宫

【标准定位】在下腹部,脐中下4寸,前正中线旁开3寸。

【毫针刺法】直刺0.8~1.2寸。

Section 7 Uterine prolapse

Combination Point Bǎi Huì—Zǐgōng.

Actions Calming the spirit and countering prolapse.

DU 20 Bǎi Huì

Position On the head, 5 cun posterior to the midpoint of the anterior hairline, and at the midpoint of the line between the two ears.

Acupuncture Insert the needle subcutaneously 0.5~0.8 cun deep and stimulate until there is a sore and distending sensation in the local area.

EX – CA 5 Zǐgōng

Position On the lower abdomen, 3 cun lateral to the anterior midline, at the level with RN 3 (zhōng jí) .

Acupuncture Insert the needle perpendicularly 0.8~1.2 cun deep.

图 3-7 百会—子宫

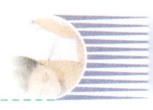

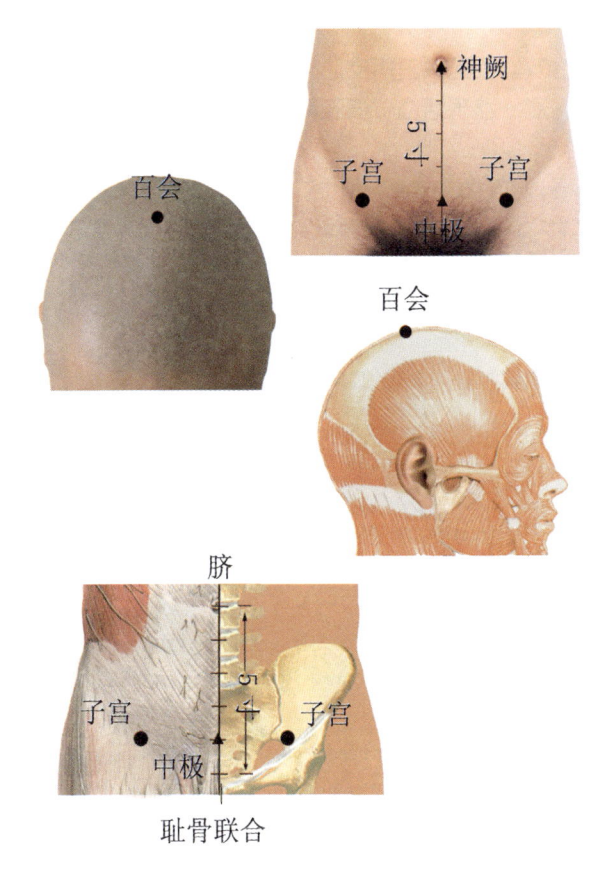

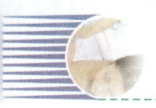

第八节　不孕症

组合穴　关元—三阴交。

功　能　益气活血，调经种子。

关元

【标准定位】在下腹部，脐中下3寸，前正中线上。

【毫针刺法】需排尿后进行针刺。直刺0.5～1.0寸，局部酸胀，可放射至外生殖器和会阴部。

三阴交

【标准定位】当足内踝尖上3寸，胫骨内侧缘后方。

【毫针刺法】直刺1.0～1.5寸。孕妇不宜针。

Section 8　Amenorrhoea

Combination Point　Guān Yuán—Sān Yīn Jiāo.

Actions　benefiting qi and Promoting blood flow, regulating menstruation and helping to pregnancy.

RN4 Guān Yuán

Position　On the lower abdomen, on the anterior midline, 3 cun inferior to the umbilicus.

Acupuncture　Insert the needle after the micturition, perpendicularly 0.5～1.0 cun deep and stimulate until there is a sore and distending sensation in the local area radiating to the genitalia.

SP 6 Sān Yīn Jiāo

Position　On the medial part of the leg, 3 cun superior to the tip of medial malleolus, posterior to the medial edge of the tibia.

Acupuncture　Insert the needle perpendicularly 0.5～1.5 cun deep and stimulate until there is a sore and numbing sensation in the local area.

图 3-8　关元—三阴交

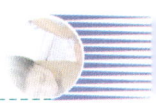

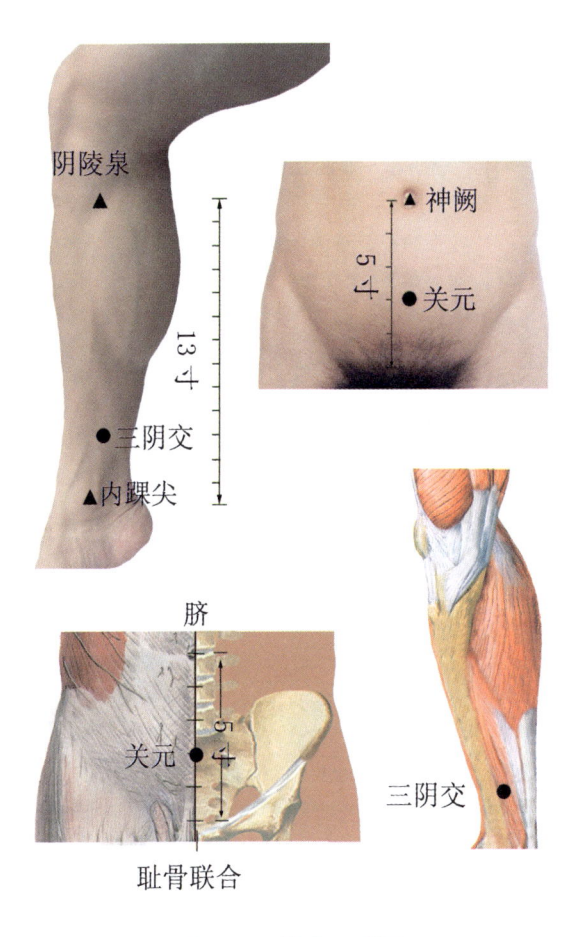

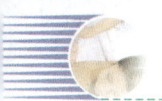

第九节 妊娠呕吐

组合穴 中脘—内关。

功 能 理气和胃,降逆止呕。

中脘

【标准定位】在上腹部,脐中上4寸,前正中线上。

【毫针刺法】直刺0.5~1.0寸,局部酸胀沉重。

内关

【标准定位】在前臂前区,腕掌侧远端横纹上2寸,掌长肌腱与桡侧腕屈肌腱之间。

【毫针刺法】直刺0.5~1.5寸,局部酸胀。

Section 9 Vomiting of pregnancy

Combination Point Zhōng Wǎn—Nèi Guān.

Actions Regulating qi and alleviating vomiting.

RN12 Zhōng Wǎn

Position On the upper abdomen, on the anterior midline, 4 cun superior to the umbilicus.

Acupuncture Insert the needle perpendicularly 0.5 ~ 1.0 cun deep and stimulate until there is a sore and distending sensation in the local area.

PC 6 Nèi Guān

Position On the palmar aspect of the forearm, 2 cun superior to the transverse crease of the wrist, between palmaris longus tendon and flexor carpi radialis tendon.

Acupuncture Insert the needle perpendicularly 0.5 ~ 1.5 cun deep and stimulate until there is a sore and numbing sensation.

图 3-9　中脘—内关

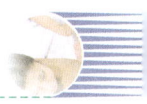

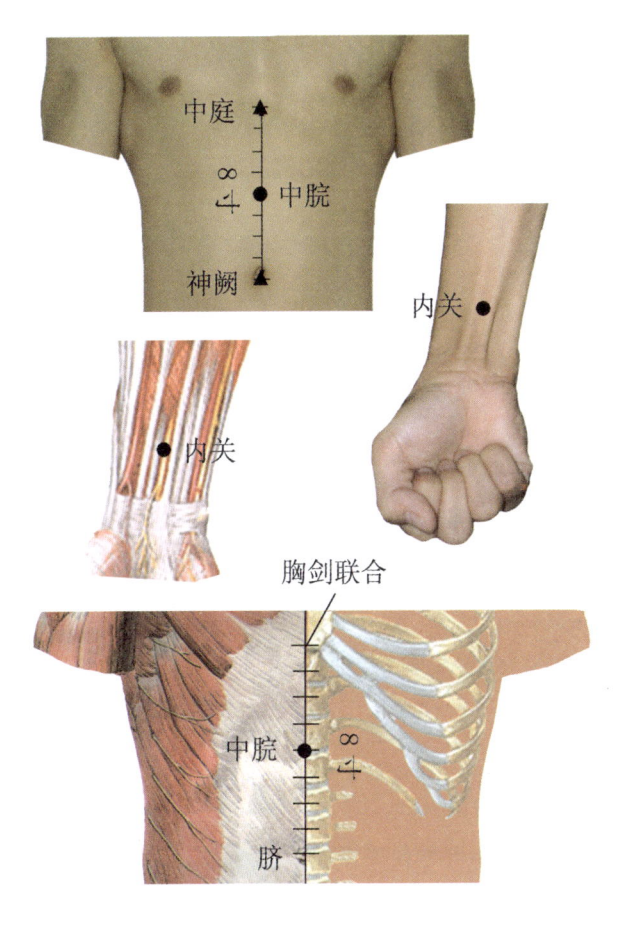

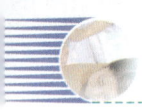

第十节　胎位不正

组合穴　至阴—足三里。

功　能　益气养血，调整胎位。

至阴

【标准定位】在足趾，小趾末节外侧，趾甲根角侧后方 0.1 寸（指寸）。

【毫针刺法】直刺 0.1～0.2 寸。

足三里

【标准定位】在小腿外侧，犊鼻（ST 35）下 3 寸，犊鼻（ST 35）与解溪（ST 41）连线上。

【毫针刺法】直刺 0.5～1.5 寸，局部酸胀。

Section 10　Malposition

Combination Point　Zhì Yīn—Zú Sān Lǐ.

Actions　Tonifying qi and nourishing blood, correcting the fetal position.

BL 67 Zhì Yīn

Position　On the lateral border of the end of small toe, 0.1 cun from the lateral corner of the nail.

Acupuncture　Insert the needle perpendicularly 0.1～0.2 cun deep.

ST36 Zú Sān Lǐ

Position　On the anterior aspect of the lower leg, 3 cun distal to ST 35 (dú bí), one finger width lateral from the anterior ridge of the tibia.

Acupuncture　Insert the needle perpendicularly 0.5～1.5 cun deep and stimulate until there is a sore and distending sensation.

图 3-10 至阴—足三里

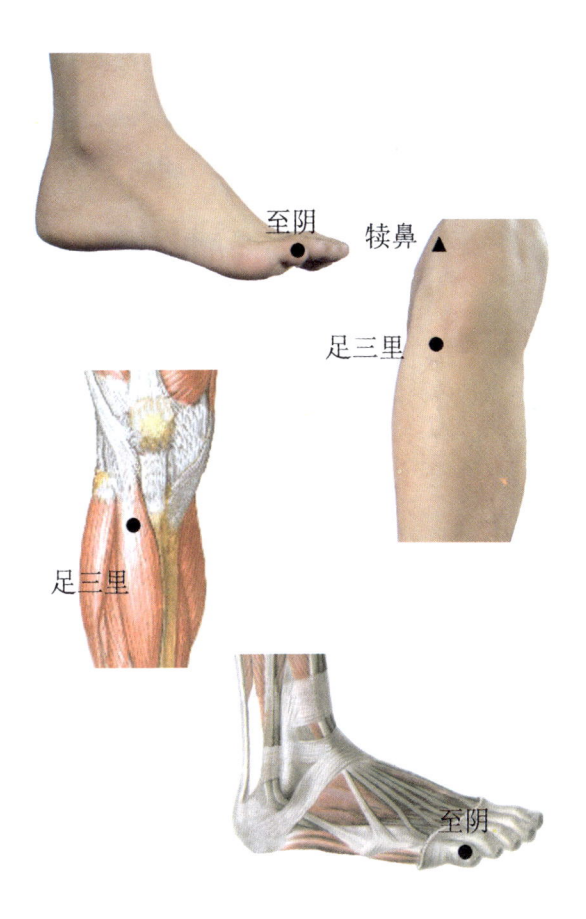

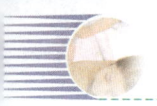

第十一节 滞 产

组合穴 合谷—三阴交。

功 能 调理气血,催产。

合谷

【标准定位】在手背,第 2 掌骨桡侧的中点处。

【毫针刺法】直刺 0.5~1.0 寸,局部酸胀。

三阴交

【标准定位】当足内踝尖上 3 寸,胫骨内侧缘后方。

【毫针刺法】直刺 1.0~1.5 寸。孕妇不宜针。

Section 11　Stagnant production

Combination Point 　Hé Gǔ—Sān Yīn Jiāo.

Actions 　Regulating qi, promoting blood flow and hastening parturition.

LI 4 Hé Gǔ

Position 　On the dorsum of the hand, between the first and second metacarpal bones, on the radial side of the middle of the second metacarpal bone.

Acupuncture 　Insert the needle perpendicularly 0.5~1.0 cun deep.

SP 6 Sān Yīn Jiāo

Position 　On the medial part of the leg, 3 cun superior to the tip of medial malleolus, posterior to the medial edge of the tibia.

Acupuncture 　Insert the needle perpendicularly 0.5~1.5 cun deep and stimulate until there is a sore and numbing sensation in the local area.

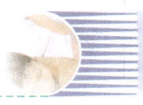

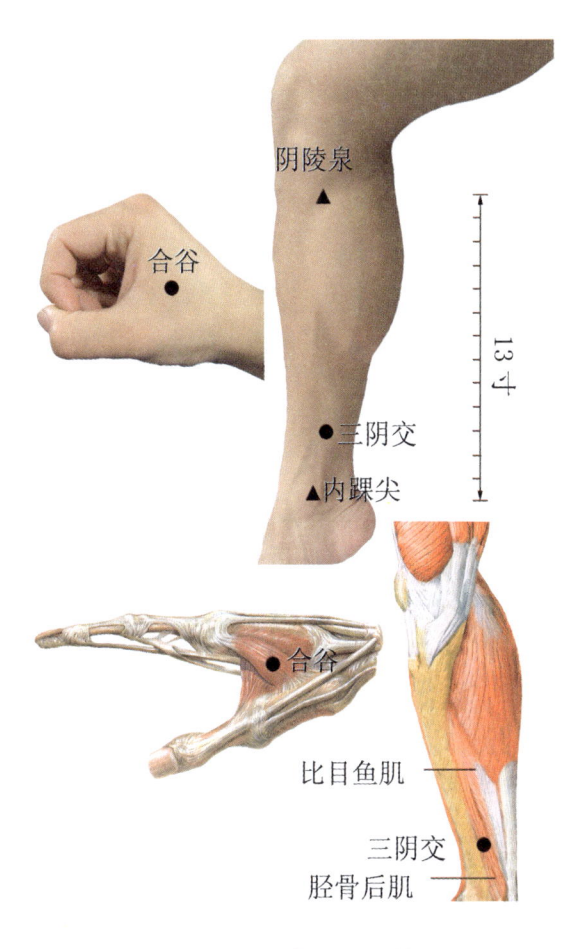

第三章 妇科、男科病证
Chapter 3 Gynecological and male diseases

阴陵泉
▲

合谷
●

13寸

● 三阴交
▲内踝尖

● 合谷

比目鱼肌
三阴交 ●
胫骨后肌

图 3-11 合谷—三阴交

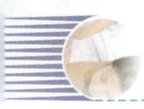

第十二节 恶露不绝

组合穴 血海—三阴交。
功 能 活血化瘀,调养胞宫。

血海
【标准定位】屈膝,在大腿内侧,髌底内侧端上2寸,当股四头肌内侧头的隆起处。
【毫针刺法】直刺1.0~2.0寸,局部酸胀。

三阴交
【标准定位】当足内踝尖上3寸,胫骨内侧缘后方。
【毫针刺法】直刺1.0~1.5寸。孕妇不宜针。

Section 12　Prolonged lochia

Combination Point　Xuè Hǎi—Sān Yīn Jiāo.

Actions　Promoting blood flow and dispelling stasis, nourishing uterus.

SP 10 Xuè Hǎi

Position　In the medial aspect of the thigh, 2 cun proximal to the medial edge of the patella, on the bulge of the medial portion of m. quadriceps femoris when the knee is flexed.

Acupuncture　Insert the needle perpendicularly 1.0~2.0 cun deep.

SP 6 Sān Yīn Jiāo

Position　On the medial part of the leg, 3 cun superior to the tip of medial malleolus, posterior to the medial edge of the tibia.

Acupuncture　Insert the needle perpendicularly 0.5~1.5 cun deep and stimulate until there is a sore and numbing sensation in the local area.

图 3-12　血海—三阴交

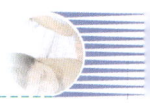

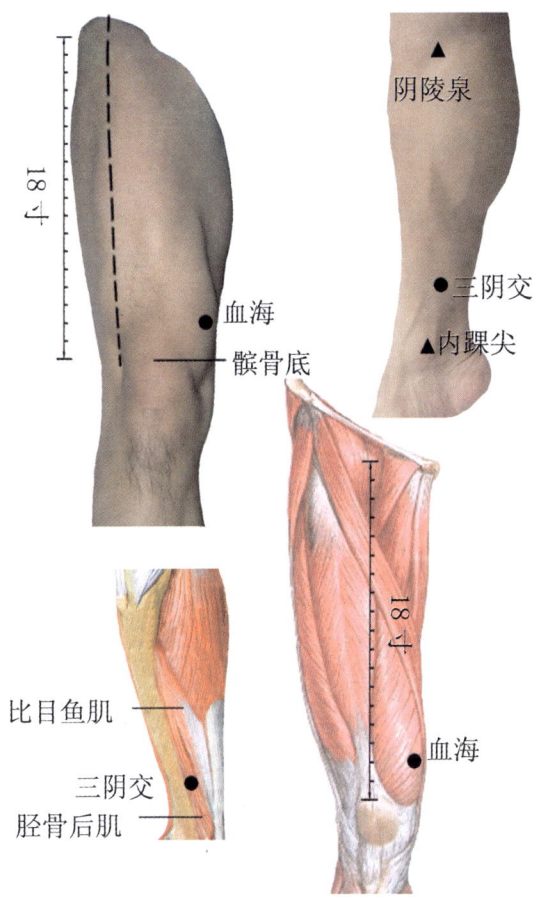

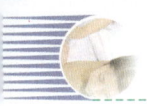

第十三节　产后乳少

组合穴　膻中—少泽。
功　能　补益气血，通乳络。

膻中

【标准定位】在胸部，当前正中线上，平第四肋间，两乳头连线的中点。

【毫针刺法】平刺 0.3~0.5 寸。

少泽

【标准定位】在手指，小指末节尺侧，距指甲根角侧上方 0.1 寸（指寸）。

【毫针刺法】直刺 0.1~0.2 寸。

Section 13　Postpartum hypogalactia

Combination Point　Tán Zhōng—Shào Zé.

Actions　Invigorating qi and blood, promoting lactation.

RN17 Tán Zhōng

Position　On the chest, on the anterior midline, at the level of the fourth intercostal space, at the midpoint between the two nipples.

Acupuncture　Insert the needle subcutaneously or obliquely 0.3~0.5 cun deep.

SI 1 Shào Zé

Position　On the ulnar side of the distal phalanx of the little finger, 0.1 cun lateral to the corner of the nail.

Acupuncture　Insert the needle 0.1~0.2 cun deep.

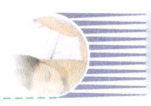

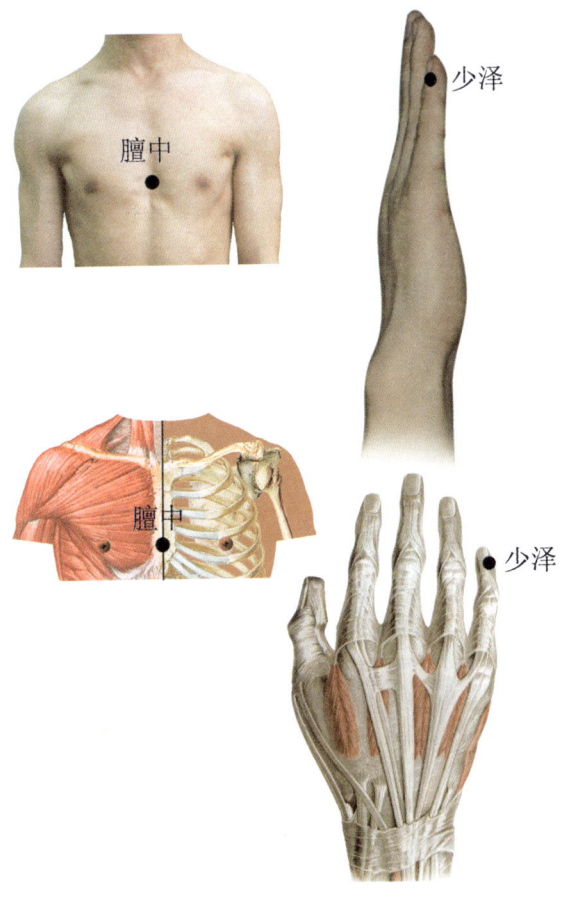

第三章 妇科、男科病证
Chapter 3　Gynecological and male diseases

图 3-13　膻中—少泽

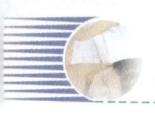

第十四节　围绝经期综合征

组合穴　神门—三阴交。
功　能　养阴安神。

神门

【标准定位】在腕前区，腕掌侧远端横纹尺侧端，尺侧腕屈肌腱的桡侧缘。

【毫针刺法】平刺 0.3~0.5 寸，局部胀痛。

三阴交

【标准定位】当足内踝尖上 3 寸，胫骨内侧缘后方。

【毫针刺法】直刺 1.0~1.5 寸。孕妇不宜针。

Section 14　Climacteric syndrome

Combination Point 　Shén Mén—Sān Yīn Jiāo.

Actions 　Nourishing Yin and calming the spirit.

HT 7 Shén Mén

Position　On the radial side of the tendon m. flexor carpi ulnaris of the transverse wrist crease.

Acupuncture　Insert the needle perpendicularly 0.3~0.5 cun deep.

SP 6 Sān Yīn Jiāo

Position　On the medial part of the leg, 3 cun superior to the tip of medial malleolus, posterior to the medial edge of the tibia.

Acupuncture　Insert the needle perpendicularly 0.5~1.5 cun deep and stimulate until there is a sore and numbing sensation in the local area.

图 3-14　神门—三阴交

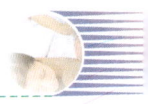

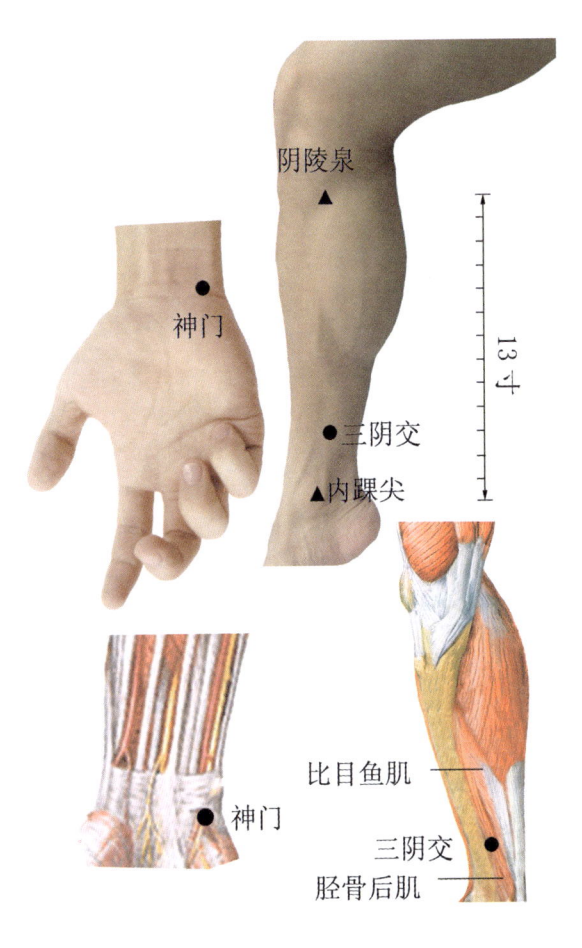

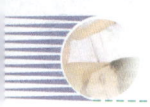

第十五节 经前期紧张综合征

组合穴 合谷—太冲。

功　能 条畅气机，镇静安神。

合谷

【标准定位】当1、2掌骨间，第2掌骨桡侧的中点

【毫针刺法】直刺0.5~1.0寸，局部酸胀。

太冲

【标准定位】当1、2跖骨间，跖骨底结合部前方凹陷中。

【毫针刺法】向上斜刺0.5~1.0，局部酸胀或麻。

Section 15　Premenstrual tension syndrome

Combination Point　Hé Gǔ— Tài Chōng.

Actions　Regulating qi and calming the spirit.

LI 4 Hé Gǔ

Position　On the dorsum of the hand, between the first and second metacarpal bones, on the radial side of the middle of the second metacarpal bone.

Acupuncture　Insert the needle perpendicularly 0.5~1.0 cun deep.

LV 3 Tài Chōng

Position　On the dorsum of the foot, in the depression proximal to the first metatarsal space.

Acupuncture　Insert the needle obliquely upwards 0.5~1.0 cun deep and stimulate until there is a sore and numbing sensation.

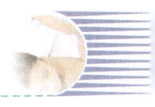

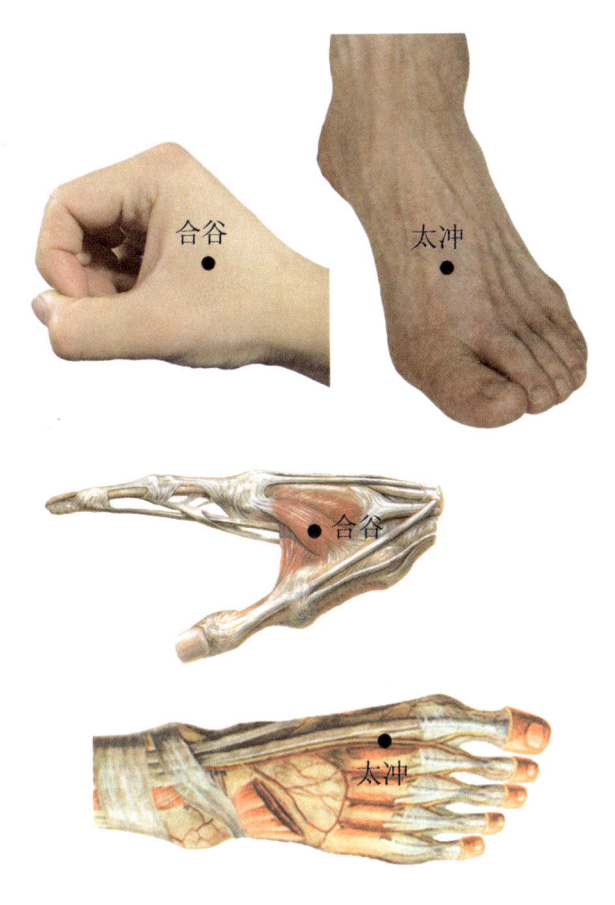

第三章　妇科、男科病证
Chapter 3　Gynecological and male diseases

图 3-15　合谷—太冲

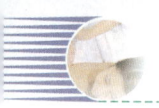

第十六节 遗 精

组合穴 关元—神门。
功 能 补益下元,安神止遗。

关元
【标准定位】在下腹部,脐中下3寸,前正中线上。
【毫针刺法】需排尿后进行针刺。直刺0.5~1.0寸,局部酸胀,可放射至外生殖器和会阴部。

神门
【标准定位】在腕前区,腕掌侧远端横纹尺侧端,尺侧腕屈肌腱的桡侧缘。
【毫针刺法】平刺0.3~0.5寸,局部胀痛。

Section 16　Seminal emission

Combination Point　Guān Yuán—Shén Mén.

Actions　Tonifying original qi and benefiting essence, calming the spirit and treating seminal emission.

RN4 Guān Yuán

Position　On the lower abdomen, on the anterior midline, 3 cun inferior to the umbilicus.

Acupuncture　Insert the needle after the micturition, perpendicularly 0.5~1.0 cun deep and stimulate until there is a sore and distending sensation in the local area radiating to the genitalia.

HT 7 Shénmén

Position　On the radial side of the tendon m. flexor carpi ulnaris of the transverse wrist crease.

Acupuncture　Insert the needle perpendicularly 0.3~0.5 cun deep.

图 3-16　关元—神门

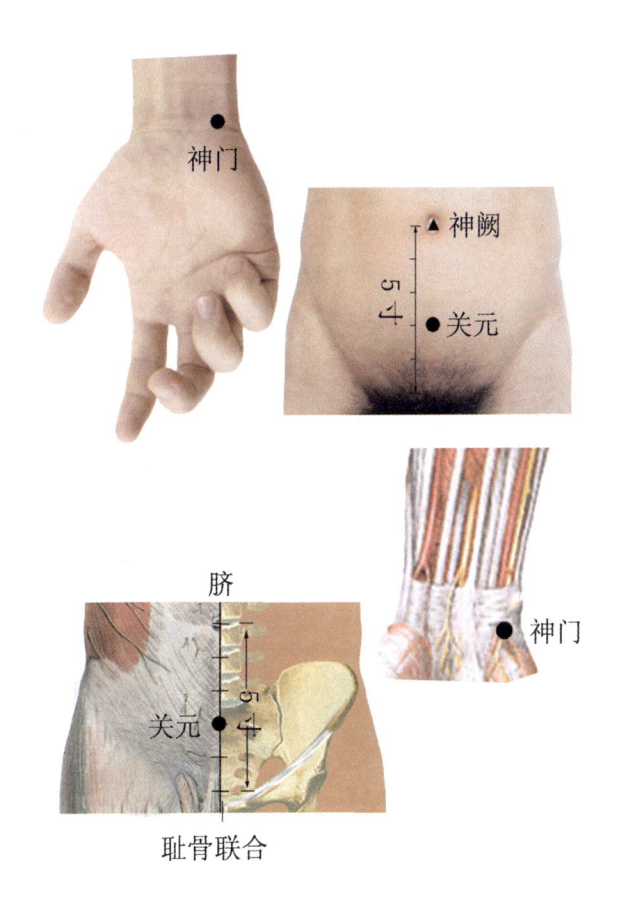

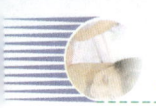

第十七节 阳 痿

组合穴 气海—关元。
功 能 大补元气,温肾助阳。

气海
【标准定位】在下腹部,脐中下1.5寸,前正中线上。
【毫针刺法】直刺0.8~1.2寸,局部酸胀,针感可向外生殖器放散。

关元
【标准定位】在下腹部,脐中下3寸,前正中线上。
【毫针刺法】需排尿后进行针刺。直刺0.5~1.0寸,局部酸胀,可放射至外生殖器和会阴部。

Section 17 Impotence

Combination Point Qì Hǎi— Guān Yuán.

Actions Tonifying original qi and benefiting essence, tonifying kidney and fortifying yang.

RN 6 Qì Hǎi

Position On the lower abdomen, on the anterior midline, 2 cun inferior to the umbilicus.

Acupuncture Insert the needle perpendicularly 0.8 ~ 1.2 cun deep and stimulate until there is a sore and distending sensation in the local area.

RN 4 Guān Yuán

Position On the lower abdomen, on the anterior midline, 3 cun inferior to the umbilicus.

Acupuncture Insert the needle perpendicularly 0.5 ~ 1.0 cun deep and stimulate until there is a sore and distending sensation in the local area radiating to the genitalia.

图 3-17　气海—关元

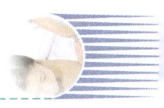

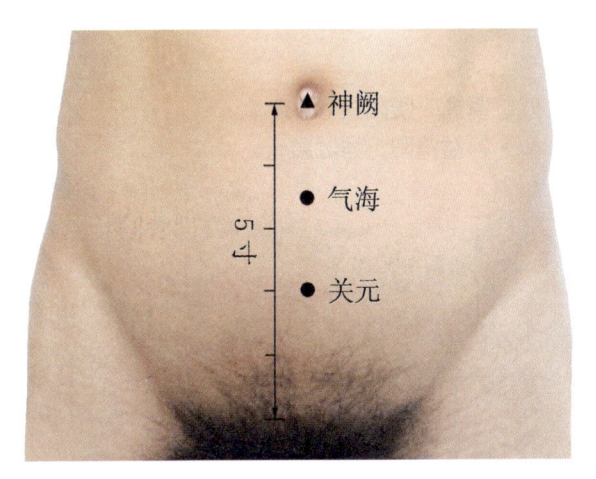

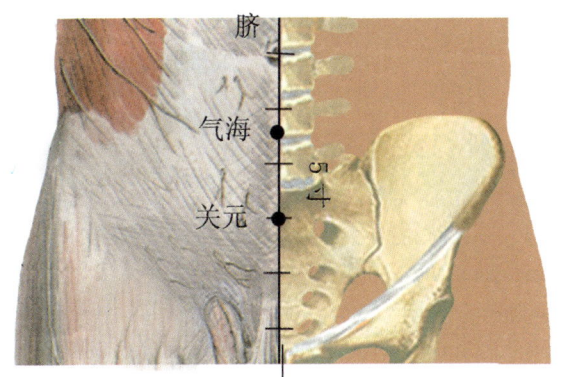

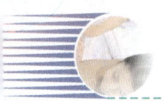

第十八节 早 泄

组合穴 肾俞—腰阳关。
功 能 补益肾阳,强壮腰脊。

肾俞
【标准定位】 在脊柱区,第2腰椎棘突下,后正中线旁开1.5寸。
【毫针刺法】 直刺0.5~0.8寸。

腰阳关
【标准定位】 在脊柱区,第4腰椎棘突下凹陷中。
【毫针刺法】 直刺或斜刺0.5~1.0寸,局部酸胀。

Section 18   Premature ejaculation

Combination Point   Shèn Shū— Yāo Yáng Guān.

Actions   Tonifying kidney and fortifying yang, strenthening lumbar region.

BL 23 Shèn Shū

Position   On the lower back, 1.5 cun lateral to the lower border of the spinous process of the second lumbar vertebra.

Acupuncture   Insert the needle perpendicularly 0.5~0.8 cun deep.

DU 3 Yāo Yáng Guān

Position   On the lumbar region, on the posterior midline, in the depression inferior to the spinous process of the fourth lumbar vertebra.

Acupuncture   Insert the needle perpendicularly or obliquely 0.5~1.0 cun deep and stimulate until there is a sore and numbing sensation in the local area radiating to the lower limbs.

图 3-18 肾俞—腰阳关

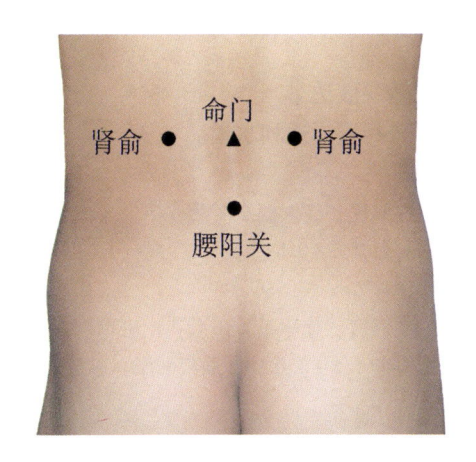

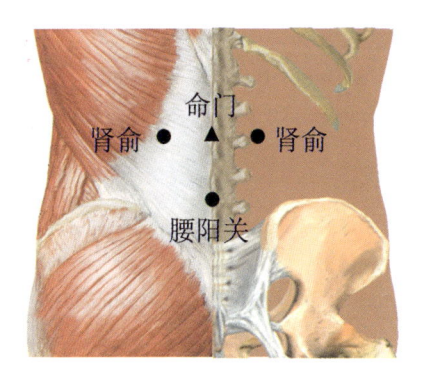

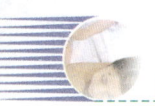

第十九节 前列腺炎

组合穴 次髎—秩边。
功 能 清热利湿,通利水道。

次髎
【标准定位】 在骶区,正对第 2 骶后孔中。
【毫针刺法】 直刺 0.5~0.8 寸。

秩边
【标准定位】 在骶区,横平第 4 骶后孔,骶正中嵴旁开 3 寸。
【毫针刺法】 直刺 1.5~3.0 寸,局部酸胀,可放射至外生殖器和会阴部。

Section 19 Prostatitis

Combination Point Cì Liáo—Zhì Biān.

Actions Transforming dampness and clearing heat, dredging the urinary tract.

BL32 Cì Liáo

Position On the sacrum, in the depression of the second posterior sacral foramen.

Acupuncture Insert the needle perpendicularly 0.5~0.8 cun deep.

BL 54 Zhì Biān

Position On the lower back, 3 cun lateral to the middle sacral creast, at the level with the fourth posterior sacral foramen.

Acupuncture Insert the needle perpendicularly obliquely 1.5~3 cun deep and stimulate until there is a sore and numbing sensation in the local area radiating to the lower abdomen.

第三章 妇科、男科病证
Chapter 3 Gynecological and male diseases

次髎

秩边

次髎

秩边

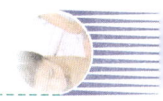

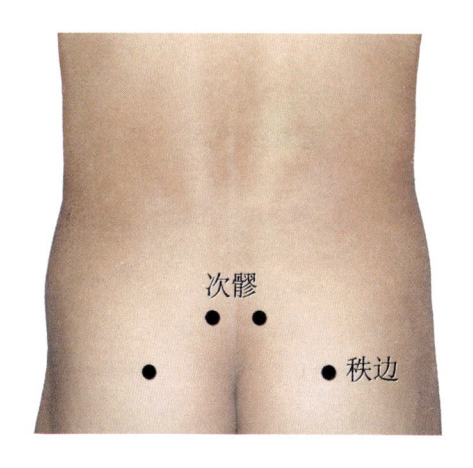

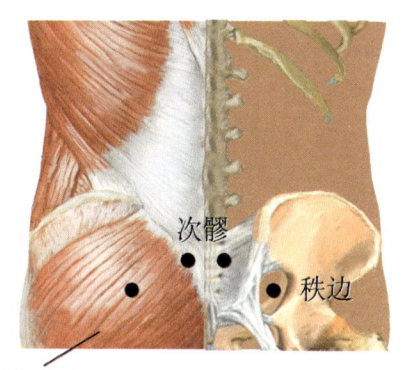

臀大肌

图3-19 次髎—秩边

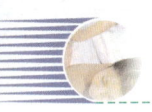

第二十节 男性不育症

组合穴 肾俞—腰阳关。

功 能 补益肾阳,强壮腰脊。

肾俞

【标准定位】 在脊柱区,第 2 腰椎棘突下,后正中线旁开 1.5 寸。

【毫针刺法】 直刺 0.5~0.8 寸。

腰阳关

【标准定位】 在脊柱区,第 4 腰椎棘突下凹陷中。

【毫针刺法】 直刺或斜刺 0.5~1.0 寸,局部酸胀。

Section 20 Male infertility

Combination Point Shèn Shū— Yāo Yáng Guān.

Actions Tonifying kidney and fortifying yang, strenthening lumbar region.

BL 23 Shèn Shū

Position On the lower back, 1.5 cun lateral to the lower border of the spinous process of the second lumbar vertebra.

Acupuncture Insert the needle perpendicularly 0.5~0.8 cun deep.

DU 3 Yāo Yáng Guān

Position On the lumbar region, on the posterior midline, in the depression inferior to the spinous process of the fourth lumbar vertebra.

Acupuncture Insert the needle perpendicularly or obliquely 0.5~1.0 cun deep and stimulate until there is a sore and numbing sensation in the local area radiating to the lower limbs.

图 3-20　肾俞—腰阳关

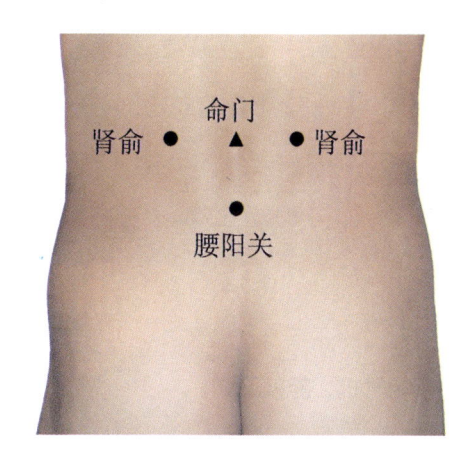

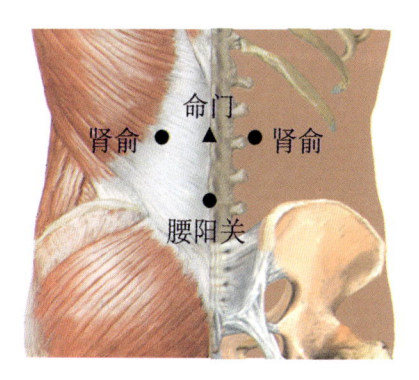

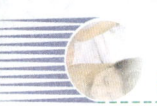

第四章 儿科病证
Chapter 4　Pediatric diseases

第一节　急惊风

组合穴　合谷—太冲。

功　能　条畅气机，豁痰开窍。

合谷

【标准定位】当1、2掌骨间，第2掌骨桡侧的中点

【毫针刺法】直刺0.5~1.0寸，局部酸胀。

太冲

【标准定位】当1、2跖骨间，跖骨底结合部前方凹陷中。

【毫针刺法】向上斜刺0.5~1.0，局部酸胀或麻。

Section 1　Acute infantile convulsion

Combination Point　Hé Gǔ— Tài Chōng.

Actions　Regulating qi and calming the spirit, dissipating phlegm and regaining consciousness.

LI 4 Hé Gǔ

Position　On the dorsum of the hand, between the first and second metacarpal bones, on the radial side of the middle of the second metacarpal bone.

Acupuncture　Insert the needle perpendicularly 0.5~1.0 cun deep.

LV 3 Tài Chōng

Position　On the dorsum of the foot, in the depression proximal to the first metatarsal space.

Acupuncture　　Insert the needle obliquely upwards 0.5 ~ 1.0 cun deep and stimulate until there is a sore and numbing sensation.

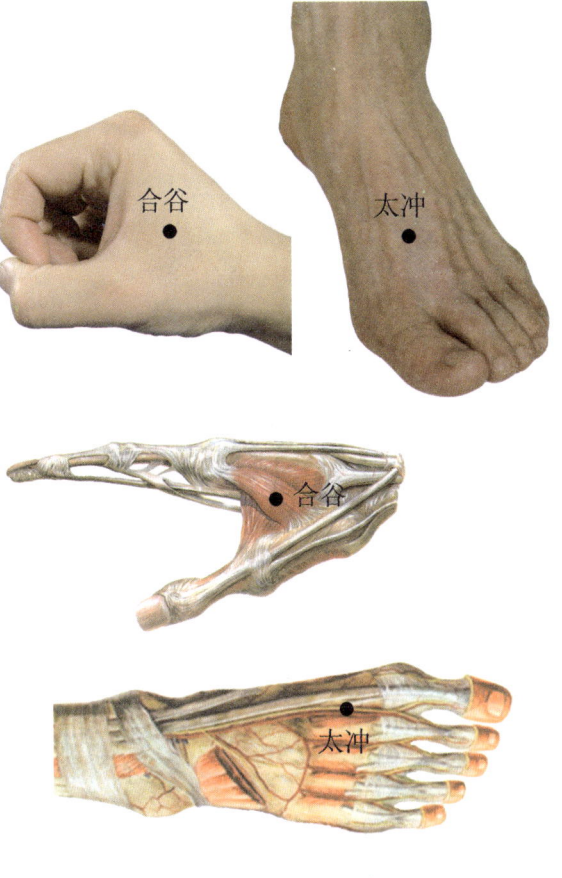

图 4-1　合谷—太冲

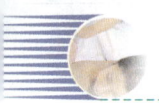

第二节 厌 食

组合穴 中脘—足三里。
功 能 理气和胃,健脾消食。

中脘

【标准定位】在上腹部,脐中上4寸,前正中线上。

【毫针刺法】直刺0.5~1.0寸,局部酸胀沉重。

足三里

【标准定位】在小腿外侧,犊鼻(ST 35)下3寸,犊鼻(ST 35)与解溪(ST 41)连线上。

【毫针刺法】直刺0.5~1.5寸,局部酸胀。

Section 2   Anorexia

Combination Point   Zhōng Wǎn—Zú Sān Lǐ.

Actions   Regulating qi and harmonizing stomach, invigorating spleen to promote digestion.

RN12 Zhōng Wǎn

Position   On the upper abdomen, on the anterior midline, 4 cun superior to the umbilicus.

Acupuncture   Insert the needle perpendicularly 0.5~1.0 cun deep and stimulate until there is a sore and distending sensation in the local area.

ST36 Zú Sān Lǐ

Position   On the anterior aspect of the lower leg, 3 cun distal to ST 35 (dú bí), one finger width lateral from the anterior ridge of the tibia.

Acupuncture   Insert the needle perpendicularly 0.5~1.5 cun deep and stimulate until there is a sore and distending sensation.

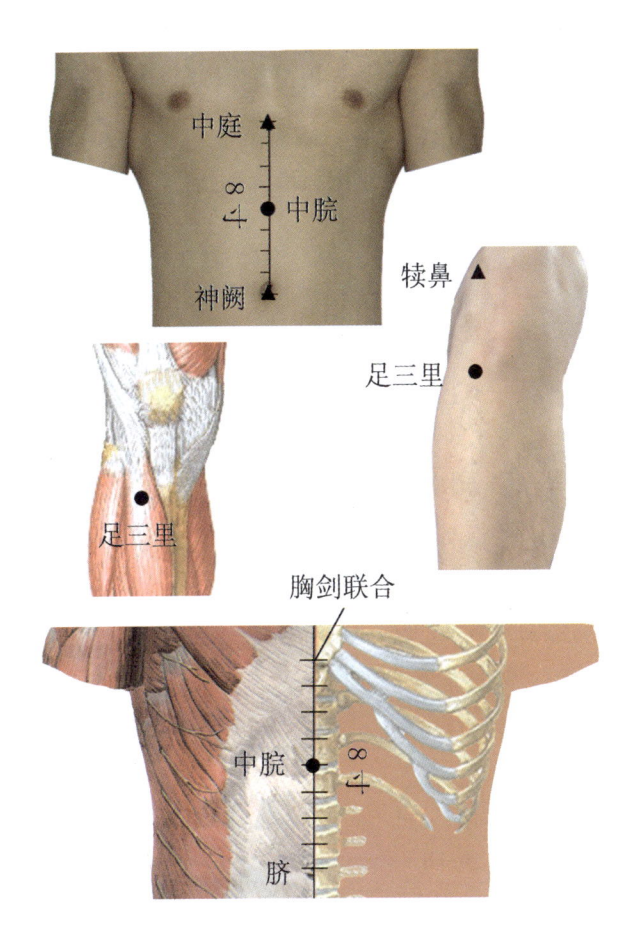

图 4-2 中脘—足三里

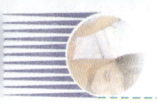

第三节 疳 证

组合穴 足三里—四缝。

功 能 健脾和胃,化积消滞。

足三里

【标准定位】在小腿外侧,犊鼻(ST 35)下3寸,犊鼻(ST 35)与解溪(ST 41)连线上。

【毫针刺法】直刺0.5~1.5寸。

四缝

【标准定位】在手指,第2至5指掌面的近侧指间关节横纹的中央,一手4穴。

【毫针刺法】点刺出血,或挤出少量淡黄色液体。

Section 3　Infantile malnutrition

Combination Point　Zú Sān Lǐ—Sì Fèng.

Actions　Invigorating spleen and harmonizing stomach to promote digestion.

ST36 Zú Sān Lǐ

Position　On the anterior aspect of the lower leg, 3 cun distal to ST 35 (dú bí), one finger width lateral from the anterior ridge of the tibia.

Acupuncture　Insert the needle perpendicularly 0.5~1.5 cun deep.

EX – UE 2 Sì Fèng

Position　A total of 8 points located on the palmar surface of the hand, in the midpoint of the transverse creases of the proximal interphalangeal joints of the index, middle, ring and little fingers.

Acupuncture　Prick with a three – edged needle to bleed, or squeeze out a small amount of yellowish viscous fluid.

第四章 儿科病证
Chapter 4　Pediatric diseases

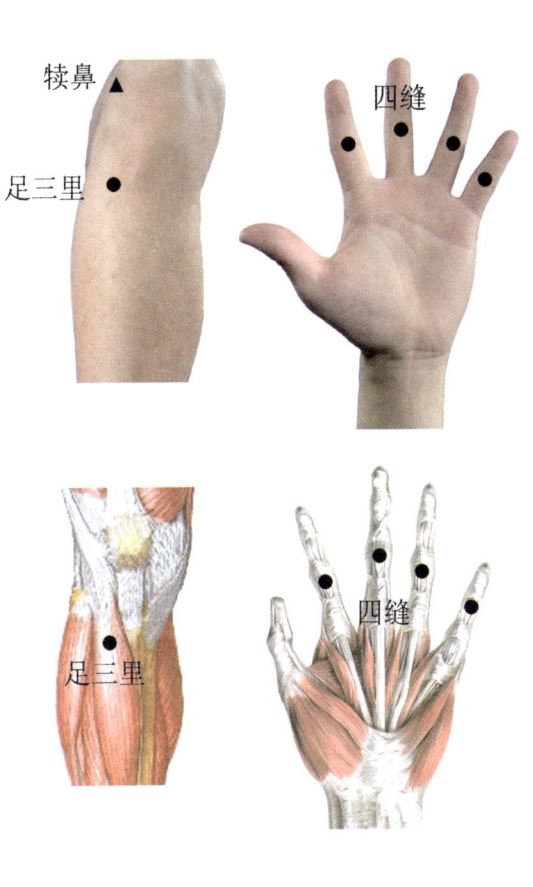

图 4-3　足三里—四缝

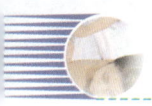

第四节 遗 尿

组合穴 中极—关元。
功 能 温肾助阳,助膀胱气化。

中极
【标准定位】在下腹部,脐中下4寸,前正中线上。
【毫针刺法】需排尿后进行针刺。直刺0.5~1.0寸,局部酸胀,可放射至外生殖器和会阴部。

关元
【标准定位】在下腹部,脐中下3寸,前正中线上。
【毫针刺法】需排尿后进行针刺。直刺0.5~1.0寸,局部酸胀,可放射至外生殖器和会阴部。

Section 4 Enuresis

Combination Point Zhōng Jí— Guān Yuán.

Actions Tonifying kidney and fortifying yang, help bladder qi transformation.

RN 3 Zhōng Jí

Position On the lower abdomen, on the anterior midline, 4 cun inferior to the umbilicus.

Acupuncture Insert the needle after the micturition, perpendicularly 0.5 ~ 1.0 cun deep and stimulate until there is a sore and distending sensation in the local area radiating to the genitalia.

RN 4 Guān Yuán

Position On the lower abdomen, on the anterior midline, 3 cun inferior to the umbilicus.

Acupuncture Insert the needle perpendicularly 0.5 ~ 1.0 cun deep and stimulate until there is a sore and distending sensation in the local area radiating to the genitalia.

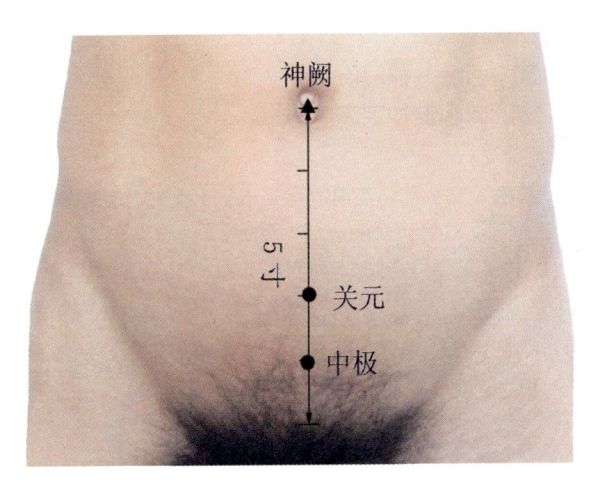

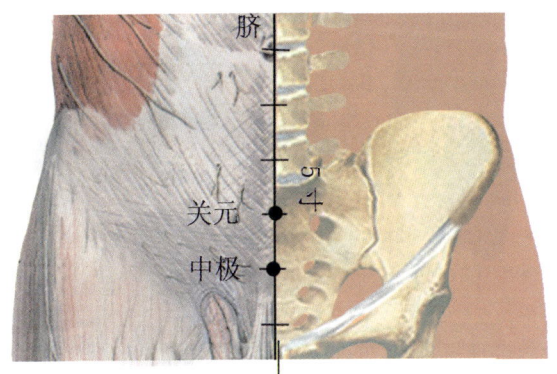

图 4-4 中极—关元

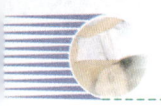

第五节 多动症

组合穴 百会—神门。

功 能 养心安神定志。

百会

【标准定位】在头部,当前发际正中直上 5 寸,或两耳尖连线的中点处。

【毫针刺法】平刺,针尖可向四周进针 0.5~0.8 寸。

神门

【标准定位】在腕前区,腕掌侧远端横纹尺侧端,尺侧腕屈肌腱的桡侧缘。

【毫针刺法】平刺 0.3~0.5 寸,局部胀痛。

Section 5 Hyperactivity

Combination Point Bǎi Huì—Shén Mén.

Actions Replenishing heart-yin to anchor the mind.

DU 20 Bǎi Huì

Position On the head, 5 cun posterior to the midpoint of the anterior hairline, and at the midpoint of the line between the two ears.

Acupuncture Insert the needle subcutaneously 0.5~0.8 cun deep.

HT 7 Shénmén

Position On the radial side of the tendon m. flexor carpi ulnaris of the transverse wrist crease.

Acupuncture Insert the needle perpendicularly 0.3~0.5 cun deep.

第四章 儿科病证
Chapter 4　Pediatric diseases

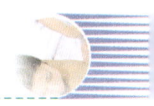

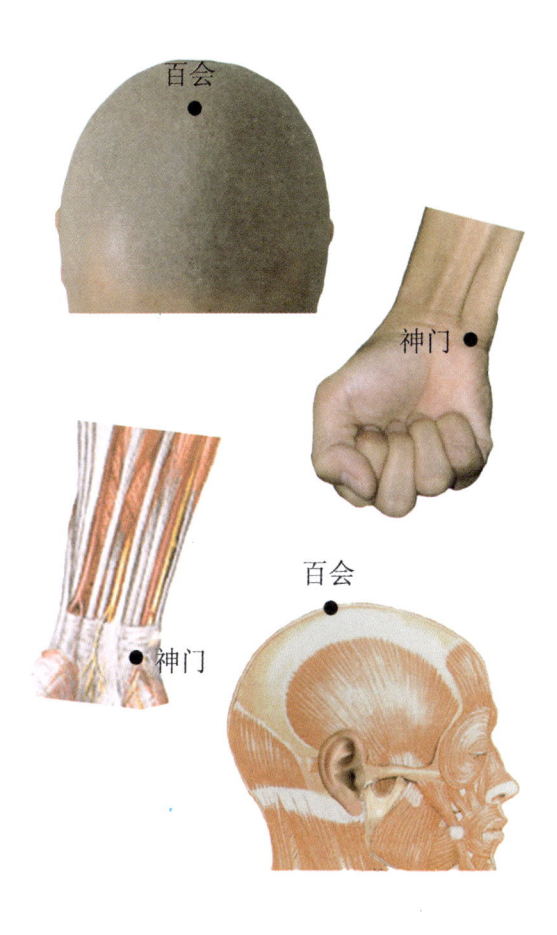

图4-5　百会—神门

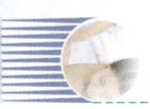

第五章 骨伤科病证
Chapter 5　Orthopedic disorders

第一节　颈椎病

组合穴　风池—天柱。

功　能　舒筋通络止痛。

风池

【标准定位】在颈后区,胸锁乳突肌上端与斜方肌上端之间的凹陷中。

【毫针刺法】向鼻尖方向斜刺 0.5~1.5 寸。

天柱

【标准定位】在颈后区,横平第 2 颈椎棘突上际,斜方肌外缘凹陷中。

【毫针刺法】直刺 0.5~0.8 寸。

Section 1　Cervical vertebra disease

Combination Point　Fēng Chí—Tiān Zhù.

Actions　Relaxing the sinews, activating the channel and alleviating pain.

GB20 Fēng Chí

Position　On the nape, in the depression between m. sternocleidomastoideus and m. trapezius.

Acupuncture　Insert the needle obliquely toward the apex nasi 0.5 ~

1.5 cun deep.

BL 10 Tiān Zhù

Position   On the neck, in the depression on the lateral border of m. trapezius, 1.3 cun lateral to the midline within the posterior hairline.

Acupuncture   Insert the needle perpendicularly 0.5 ~ 0.8 cun deep.

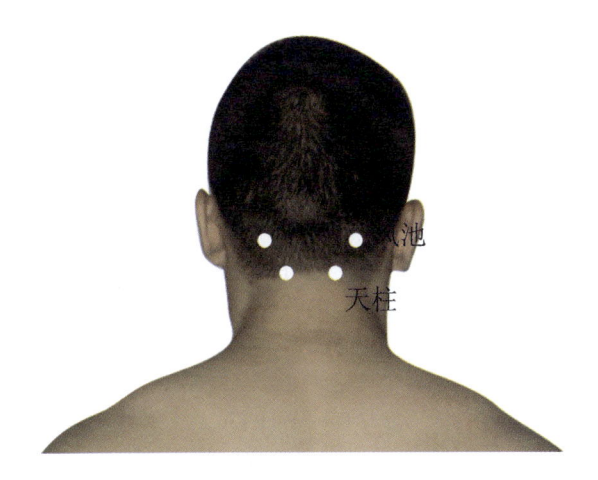

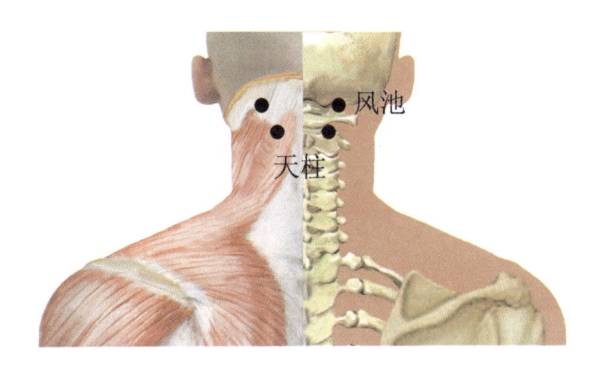

图 5-1　风池—天柱

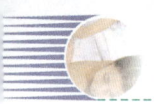

第二节 落 枕

组合穴 风池—肩井。

功 能 祛风解表,舒筋止痛。

风池

【标准定位】枕骨之下,胸锁乳突肌上端与斜方肌上端之间的凹陷中。

【毫针刺法】向对侧或同侧口角方向斜刺0.5~1.5寸。

肩井

【标准定位】在肩胛区,第7颈椎棘突与肩峰最外侧点连线的中点。

【毫针刺法】直刺或向四周斜刺0.5~0.8寸。

Section 2 Have a stiff neck

Combination Point Fēng Fǔ— Fēng Chí.

Actions Releasing the exterior and expelling wind, relaxing the sinews and alleviating pain.

GB20 Fēng Chí

Position On the back of the neck, 0.5 cun superior to the midpoint of the posterior hairline, in the depression between m. trapezius of both sides.

Acupuncture Insert the needle obliquely towards the lower jaw 0.5~1.5 cun deep.

GB 21 Jiānjǐng

Position On the shoulder, at the midpoint of the line connecting DU 14 (dà zhuī) and the acromion end of the clavicle.

Acupuncture Insert the needle subcutaneously 0.5~0.8 cun deep.

第五章 骨伤科病证
Chapter 5 Orthopedic disorders

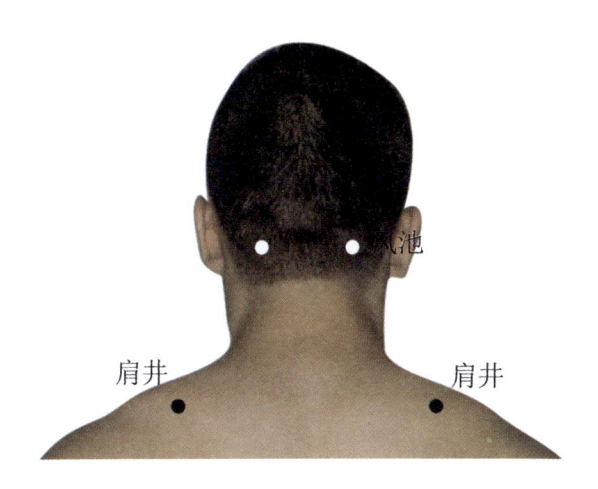

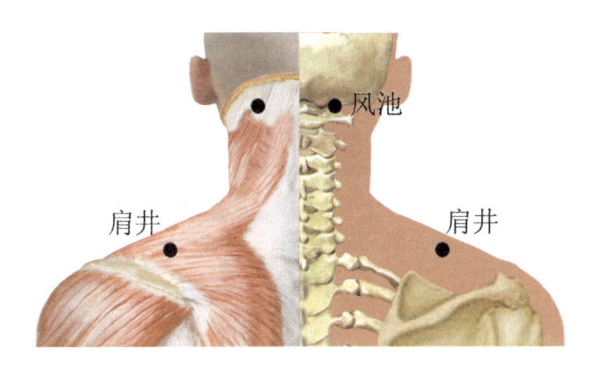

图 5-2 风池—肩井

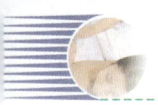

第三节　肩关节周围炎

组合穴　肩髃—肩髎。
功　能　通利关节，祛风除湿。

肩髃
【标准定位】在肩峰前下方，当肩峰与肱骨大结节之间凹陷处。
【毫针刺法】直刺1~1.5寸，局部酸胀。

肩髎
【标准定位】肩峰角与肱骨大结节两骨间凹陷中。
【毫针刺法】直刺1~1.5寸，局部酸胀。

Section 3　Periarthritis of shoulder

Combination Point　Jiān Yú— Jiān Liáo.

Actions　Dispelling wind and eliminating dampness and benefiting the joint.

LI 15 Jiān Yú

Position　In the anterior and inferior aspect of the acromion, in the depression between the acromion and the greater tubercle of the humerus.

Acupuncture　Insert the needle perpendicularly 1~1.5cun deep.

SJ 14 Jiān Liáo

Position　On the shoulder, posterior to LI 15 (jiān yú), when the arm is abducted, in the depression posterior and inferior to the acromion.

Acupuncture　Insert the needle perpendicularly 1~1.5 cun deep and stimulate until there is a sore and distending sensation.

第五章　骨伤科病证
Chapter 5　Orthopedic disorders

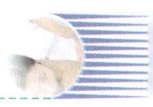

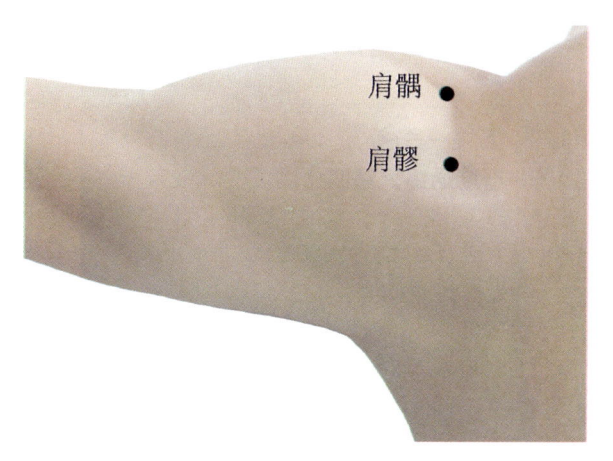

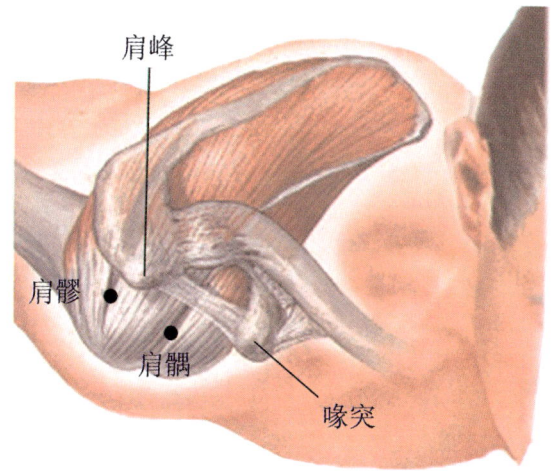

图 5-3　肩髃—肩髎

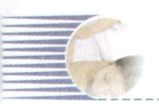

第四节 颞下颌关节功能紊乱综合征

组合穴 下关—合谷。

功 能 舒筋通络,活血止痛。

下关

【标准定位】当颧弓与下颌切迹所形成的凹陷处。

【毫针刺法】直刺 0.8~1.2 寸。

合谷

【标准定位】在手背,第1、2掌骨间,第2掌骨桡侧的中点处。

【毫针刺法】直刺 0.5~1.0 寸。

Section 4 Temporomandibular joint dysfunction syndrome

Combination Point Xià Guān—Hé Gǔ.

Actions Relaxing the sinews and activating the channel, promoting blood circulation and alleviating pain.

ST 7 Xià Guān

Position In the depression between the zygomatic arch and mandibular notch in front of the ear.

Acupuncture Insert the needle perpendicularly 0.8~1.2 cun deep.

LI 4 Hé Gǔ

Position On the dorsum of the hand, between the first and second metacarpal bones, on the radial side of the middle of the second metacarpal bone.

Acupuncture Insert the needle perpendicularly 0.5~1.0 cun deep.

第五章　骨伤科病证
Chapter 5　Orthopedic disorders

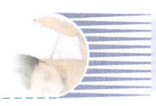

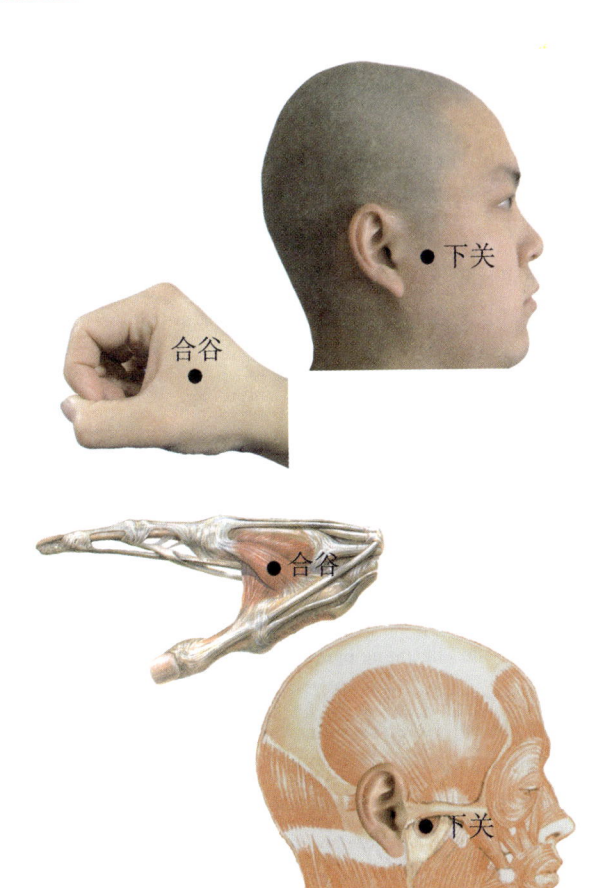

图 5-4　下关—合谷

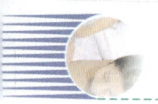

第五节 肱骨外上髁炎

组合穴 曲池—合谷。

功 能 舒筋通络,活血止痛。

曲池
【标准定位】尺泽与肱骨外上髁上连线的中点处。

【毫针刺法】直刺 1.0~2.0 寸。局部酸胀。

合谷
【标准定位】在手背,第 1、2 掌骨间,第 2 掌骨桡侧的中点处。

【毫针刺法】直刺 0.5~1.0 寸。

Section 5　External humeral epicondylitis

Combination Point　Qǔ Chí—Hé Gǔ.

Actions　Relaxing the sinews and activating the channel, promoting blood circulation and alleviating pain.

LI 11 Qǔ Chí

Position　In the depression of the radial side of the transverse cubital crease when elbow flexed.

Acupuncture　Insert the needle perpendicularly 1.0~1.5 cun deep and stimulate until there is a sore and numbing sensation in the local area.

LI 4 Hé Gǔ

Position　On the dorsum of the hand, between the first and second metacarpal bones, on the radial side of the middle of the second metacarpal bone.

Acupuncture　Insert the needle perpendicularly 0.5~1.0 cun deep.

第五章　骨伤科病证
Chapter 5　Orthopedic disorders

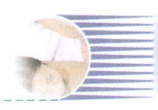

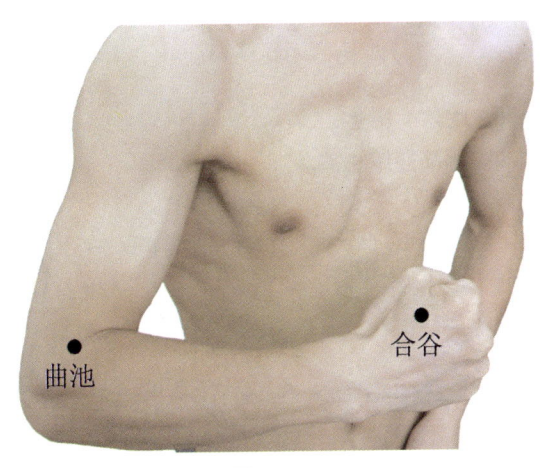

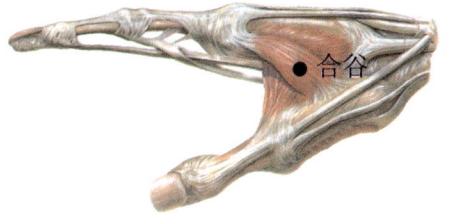

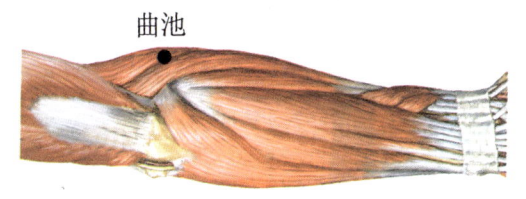

图 5-5　曲池—合谷

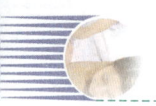

第六节 跟痛症

组合穴　申脉—照海。
功　能　舒筋通络止痛。

申脉

【标准定位】在足外侧部,外踝直下方凹陷中。
【毫针刺法】直刺或略下斜刺 0.2~0.3 寸,局部酸胀。

照海

【标准定位】在足内侧,内踝尖下方凹陷处。
【毫针刺法】直刺 0.5~0.8 寸,局部酸麻,可扩散至整个踝部。

Section 6　Heel pain

Combination Point　Shēn Mài— Zhào Hǎi.

Actions　Relaxing the sinews and activating the channel and alleviating pain.

BL 62 Shēn Mài

Position　On the lateral side of the foot, in the depression inferior to the external malleolus.

Acupuncture　Insert the needle perpendicularly 0.2~0.3 cun deep and stimulate until there is a sore and numbing sensation in the local area.

KI 6 Zhào Hǎi

Position　On the medial side of the foot, in the depression inferior to the tip of the medial malleous.

Acupuncture　Insert the needle perpendicularly 0.5~0.8 cun deep and stimulate until there is a sore and numbing sensation in the local area spreading in the ankle.

第五章 骨伤科病证
Chapter 5　Orthopedic disorders

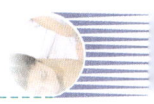

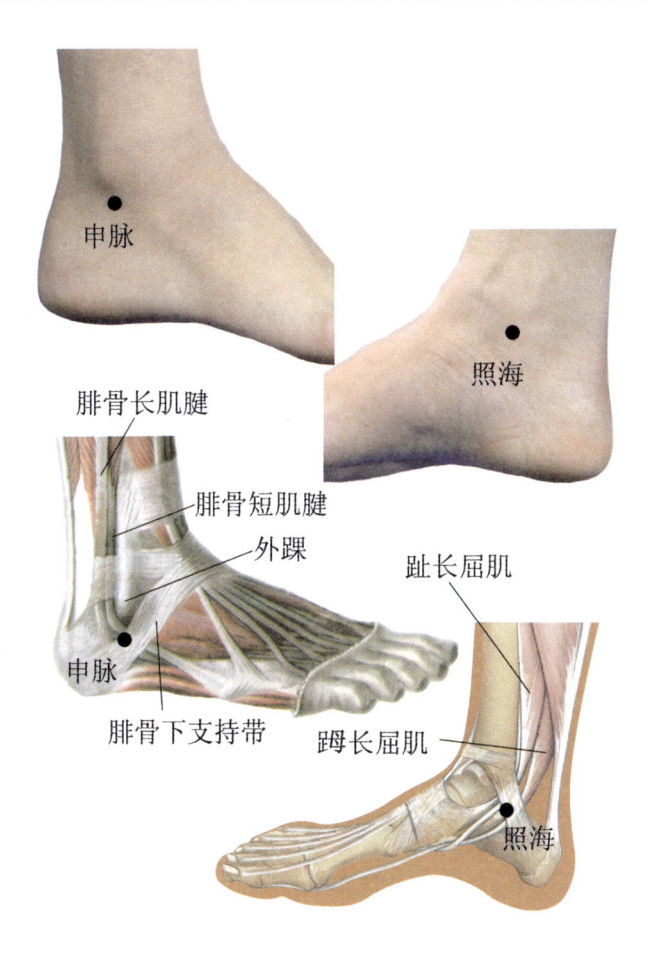

图 5-6　申脉—照海

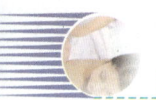

第七节 扭 伤

1. 颈部

组合穴　风池—天柱。

功　能　舒筋通络止痛。

风池

【标准定位】在颈后区,胸锁乳突肌上端与斜方肌上端之间的凹陷中。

【毫针刺法】向鼻尖方向斜刺 0.5~1.5 寸。

天柱

【标准定位】在颈后区,横平第 2 颈椎棘突上际,斜方肌外缘凹陷中。

【毫针刺法】直刺 0.5~0.8 寸。

Section 7　Sprain

1. Neck

Combination Point　Fēng Chí—Tiān Zhù.

Actions　Relaxing the sinews and activating the channel and alleviating pain.

GB20 Fēng Chí

Position　On the nape, in the depression between m. sternocleidomastoideus and m. trapezius.

Acupuncture　Insert the needle obliquely toward the apex nasi 0.5~1.5 cun deep.

BL 10 Tiān Zhù

Position　On the neck, in the depression on the lateral border of m. trapezius, 1.3 cun lateral to the midline within the posterior hairline.

Acupuncture　Insert the needle perpendicularly 0.5~0.8 cun deep.

第五章 骨伤科病证
Chapter 5 Orthopedic disorders

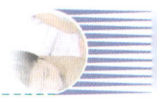

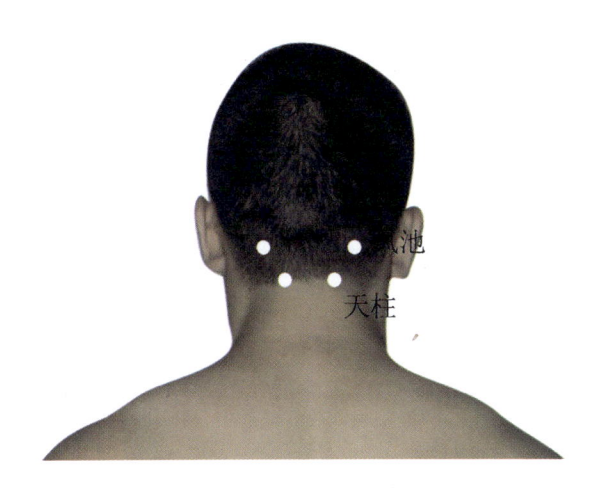

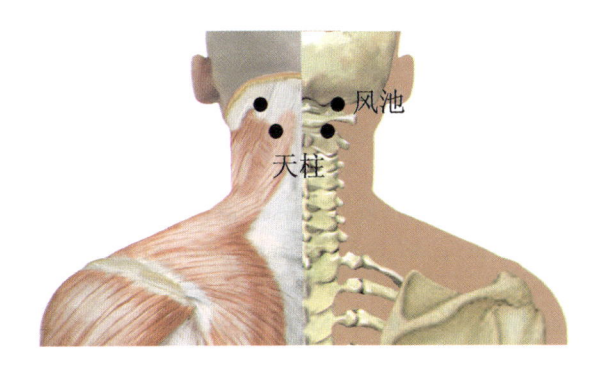

图 5-7-1 风池—天柱

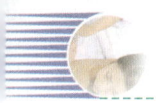

2. 肩部

组合穴 肩髃—肩髎。

功 能 舒筋通络止痛。

肩髃

【标准定位】在肩峰前下方,当肩峰与肱骨大结节之间凹陷处。

【毫针刺法】直刺 1~1.5 寸,局部酸胀。

肩髎

【标准定位】在三角肌区,肩峰角与肱骨大结节两骨间凹陷中。

【毫针刺法】直刺 1~1.5 寸,局部酸胀。

2. Shoulder

Combination Point Jiān Yú— Jiān Liáo.

Actions Relaxing the sinews and activating the channel and alleviating pain.

LI 15 Jiān Yú

Position In the anterior and inferior aspect of the acromion, in the depression between the acromion and the greater tubercle of the humerus.

Acupuncture Insert the needle perpendicularly 1~1.5cun deep and stimulate until there is a sore and distending sensation.

SJ 14 Jiān Liáo

Position On the shoulder, posterior to LI 15 (jiān yú), when the arm is abducted, in the depression posterior and inferior to the acromion.

Acupuncture Insert the needle perpendicularly 1~1.5 cun deep and stimulate until there is a sore and distending sensation.

第五章 骨伤科病证
Chapter 5 Orthopedic disorders

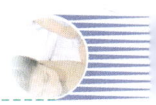

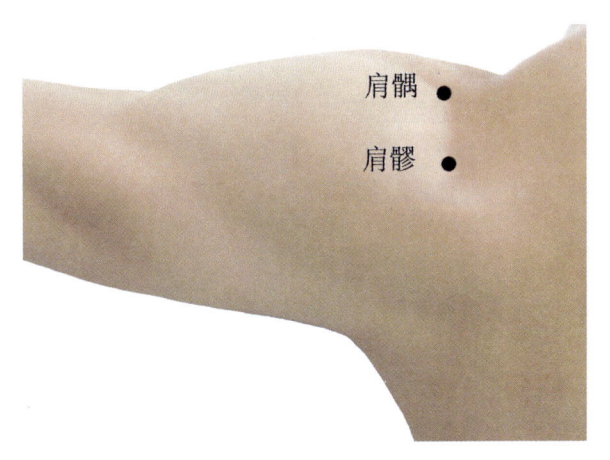

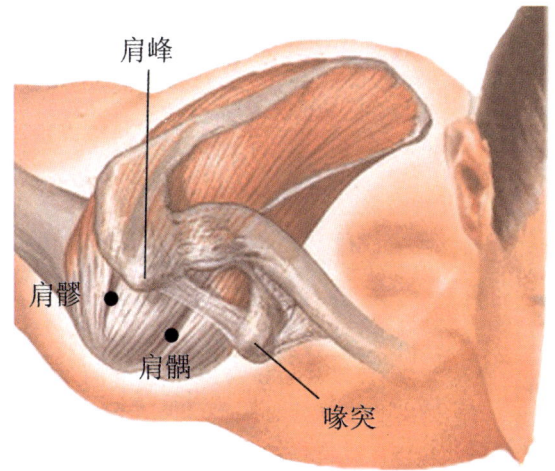

图 5-7-2　肩髃—肩髎

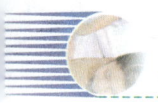

3. 肘部

组合穴　臂臑—曲池。

功　能　舒筋通络止痛。

臂臑

【标准定位】在臂部,曲池上7寸,三角肌前缘处。

【毫针刺法】直刺0.5~1寸,局部酸胀。

曲池

【标准定位】尺泽与肱骨外上髁上连线的中点处。

【毫针刺法】直刺1.0~2.0寸。局部酸胀。

3. Elbow

Combination Point　Bì Nào— Qǔ Chí.

Actions　Relaxing the sinews and activating the channel and alleviating pain.

LI 14 Bì Nào

Position　On the lateral side of the upper arm, 7 cun proximal to LI 11 (qǔ chí) on the line connecting LI 11 (qǔ chí) and LI 15 (jiān yú), in the depression formed by the distal insertion of the m. deltoideus and m. brachialis.

Acupuncture　Insert the needle perpendicularly 0.5~1 cun deep and stimulate until there is a sore and numbing sensation in the local area radiating to the forearm.

LI 11 Qǔ Chí

Position　In the depression of the radial side of the transverse cubital crease when elbow flexed.

Acupuncture　Insert the needle perpendicularly 1.0~1.5 cun deep and stimulate until there is a sore and numbing sensation in the local area radiating to the forearm.

第五章 骨伤科病证
Chapter 5　Orthopedic disorders

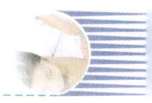

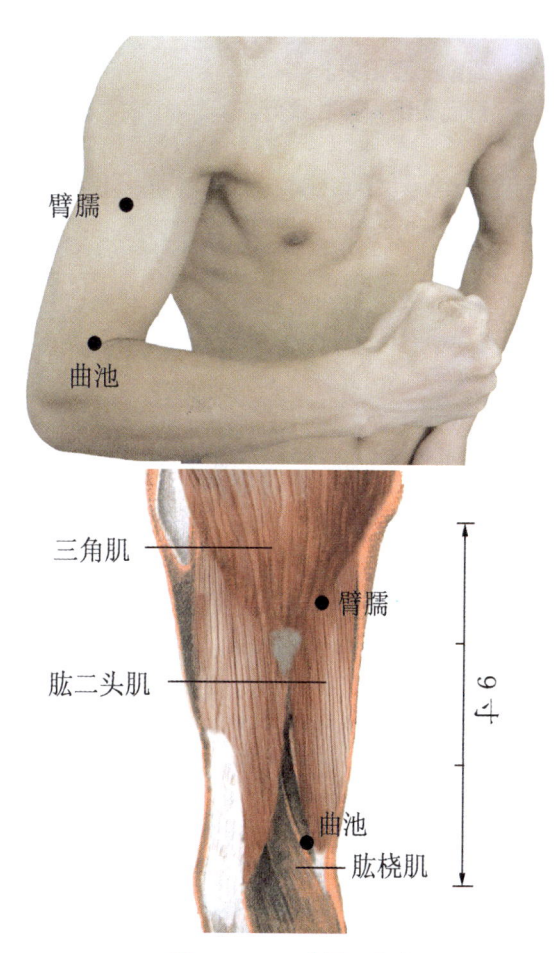

图 5-7-3　臂臑—曲池

4. 腰部

组合穴 肾俞—腰阳关。

功 能 舒筋通络,强壮腰脊。

肾俞

【标准定位】在脊柱区,第2腰椎棘突下,后正中线旁开1.5寸。

【毫针刺法】直刺0.5~0.8寸。

腰阳关

【标准定位】在脊柱区,第4腰椎棘突下凹陷中。

【毫针刺法】直刺或斜刺0.5~1.0寸,局部酸胀。

4. Lumbar

Combination Point Shèn Shū— Yāo Yáng Guān.

Actions Relaxing the sinews and activating the channel, alleviating pain and strenthens lumbar region.

BL 23 Shèn Shū

Position On the lower back, 1.5 cun lateral to the lower border of the spinous process of the second lumbar vertebra.

Acupuncture Insert the needle perpendicularly 0.5~0.8 cun deep.

DU 3 Yāo Yáng Guān

Position On the lumbar region, on the posterior midline, in the depression inferior to the spinous process of the fourth lumbar vertebra.

Acupuncture Insert the needle perpendicularly or obliquely 0.5~1.0 cun deep and stimulate until there is a sore and numbing sensation in the local area radiating to the lower limbs.

第五章　骨伤科病证
Chapter 5　Orthopedic disorders

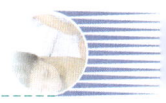

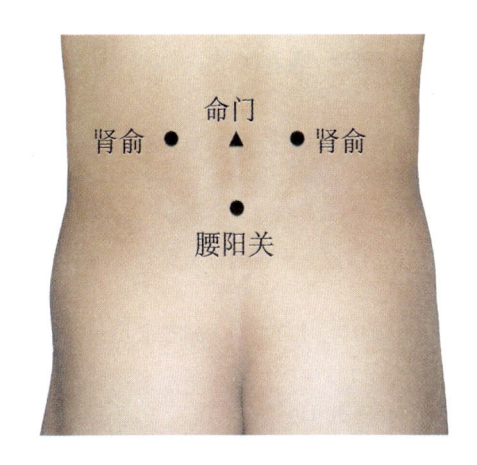

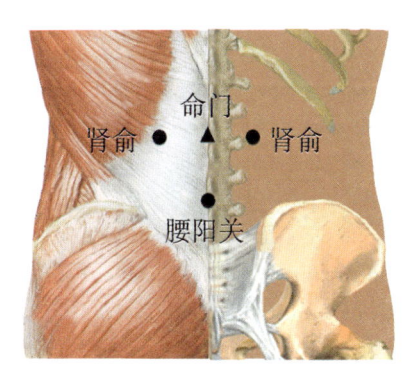

图 5-7-4　肾俞—腰阳关

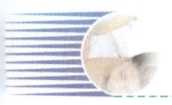

5. 髋部

组合穴　居髎—伏兔。

功　能　强壮腰膝，通利关节。

居髎

【标准定位】在髂前上棘与股骨大转子高点连线的中点处。

【毫针刺法】直刺1～1.5寸。

伏兔

【标准定位】在大腿前面，当髂前上棘与髌底外侧端的连线上，髌底上6寸。

【毫针刺法】直刺0.8～1.2寸，局部酸胀。

5. Hip

Combination Point　Jū Liáo— Fú Tù.

Actions　Strenthening lumbar region, activating the channel and benefits joints.

GB 29 Jū Liáo

Position　On the hip, at the midpoint of the line connecting the anterior superior iliac spine and the great trochanter of the femur.

Acupuncture　Insert the needle perpendicularly 1～1.5 cun deep.

ST 32 Fú Tù

Position　On the anterior aspect of the thigh, on the line connecting the anterior superior iliac spine and lateral end of the patella, 6 cun proximal to the superior border of patella.

Acupuncture　Insert the needle perpendicularly 0.8～1.2 cun deep and stimulate until there is a sore and numbing sensation.

第五章 骨伤科病证
Chapter 5　Orthopedic disorders

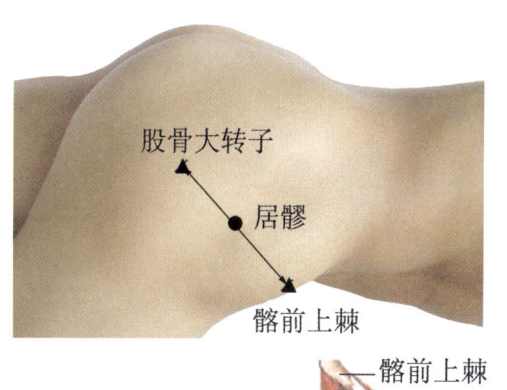

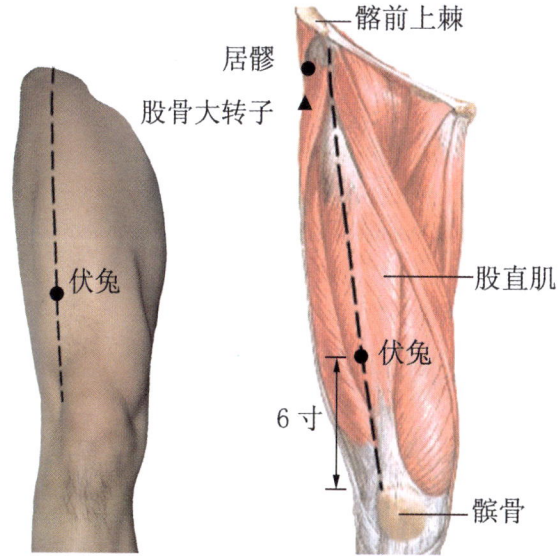

图 5-7-5　居髎—伏兔

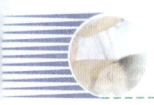

6. 膝部

组合穴 梁丘—血海。

功 能 舒筋通络止痛。

血海

【标准定位】屈膝,在大腿内侧,髌底内侧端上2寸,当股四头肌内侧头的隆起处。

【毫针刺法】直刺1.0~2.0寸,局部酸胀。

梁丘

【标准定位】在髂前上棘与髌骨底外缘连线上,当髌底上2寸处。

【毫针刺法】直刺1.0~1.5寸。

6. Knees

Combination Point Xuè Hǎi— Liáng Qiū.

Actions Relaxing the sinews, activates the channel and alleviating pain.

SP 10 Xuè Hǎi

Position In the medial aspect of the thigh, 2 cun proximal to the medial edge of the patella, on the bulge of the medial portion of m. quadriceps femoris when the knee is flexed.

Acupuncture Insert the needle perpendicularly 1.0 ~ 2.0 cun deep and stimulate until there is a sore and numbing sensation.

ST 34 Liáng Qiū

Position On the anterior aspect of the thigh, on the line connecting the anterior superior iliac spine and lateral end of the patella, 2 cun proximal to the patella when the knee is bent.

Acupuncture Insert the needle perpendicularly 1.0 ~ 1.5 cun deep.

第五章 骨伤科病证
Chapter 5 Orthopedic disorders

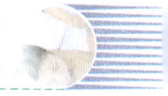

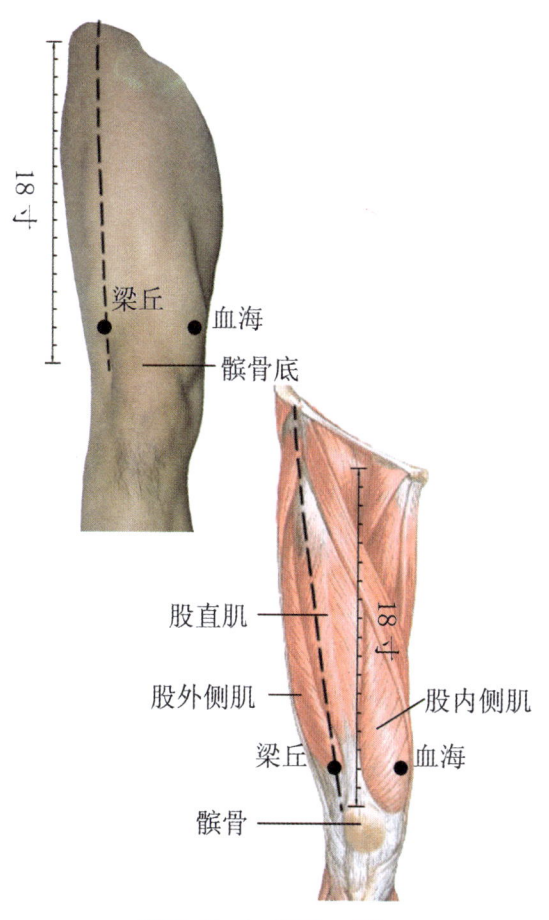

图 5-7-6 梁丘—血海

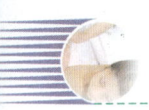

第六章 皮肤科疾病
Chapter 6　Dermatology diseases

第一节　神经性皮炎

组合穴　合谷—血海。

功　能　活血化瘀，疏风止痛。

合谷

【标准定位】在手背，第1、2掌骨间，第2掌骨桡侧的中点处。

【毫针刺法】直刺0.5~1.0寸。

血海

【标准定位】在大腿内侧，髌底内侧端上2寸。

【毫针刺法】直刺1.0~2.0寸。

Section 1　Neurodermatitis

Combination Point　Xuè Hǎi— Liáng Qiū.

Actions　Promoting blood flow and dispelling stasis, dispelling wind and alleviating pain.

LI 4 Hé Gǔ

Position　On the dorsum of the hand, between the first and second metacarpal bones, on the radial side of the middle of the second metacarpal bone.

Acupuncture　Insert the needle perpendicularly 0.5~1.0 cun deep.

SP 10 Xuè Hǎi

Position　In the medial aspect of the thigh, 2 cun proximal to the medial edge of the patella, on the bulge of the medial portion of m. quadriceps femoris when the knee is flexed.

Acupuncture　Insert the needle perpendicularly 1.0~2.0 cun deep.

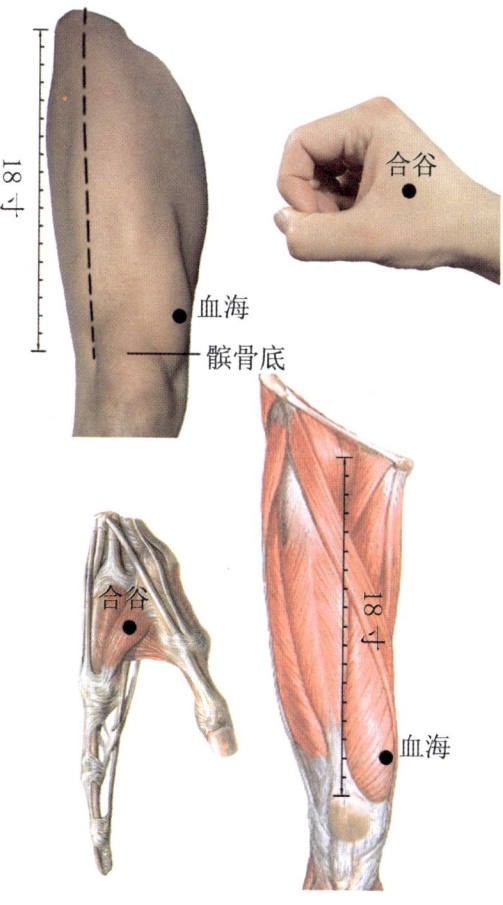

图 6-1　合谷—血海

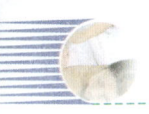

第二节 皮肤瘙痒症

组合穴 三阴交—合谷。

功 能 滋阴清热，疏风止痒。

三阴交

【标准定位】当足内踝尖上3寸，胫骨内侧缘后方。

【毫针刺法】直刺1.0~1.5寸。孕妇不宜针。

合谷

【标准定位】在手背，第2掌骨桡侧的中点处。

【毫针刺法】直刺1.0~2.0寸。局部酸胀。

Section 2　Cutaneous pruritus

Combination Point　Sān Yīn Jiāo— Hé Gǔ.

Actions　Clearing heat and nourishing yin, expelling wind and relieving itching.

SP 6 Sān Yīn Jiāo

Position　On the medial part of the leg, 3 cun superior to the tip of medial malleolus, posterior to the medial edge of the tibia.

Acupuncture　Insert the needle perpendicularly 1.0 ~ 1.5 cun deep and stimulate until there is a sore and numbing sensation in the local area.

LI 4 Hé Gǔ

Position　On the dorsum of the hand, between the first and second metacarpal bones, on the radial side of the middle of the second metacarpal bone.

Acupuncture　Insert the needle perpendicularly 1.0 ~ 1.5cun deep and stimulte until there is a sore and numbing sensation in the local area radiating to the elbow, shoulder and face.

第六章　皮肤科疾病
Chapter 6　Dermatology diseases

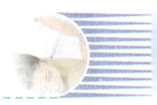

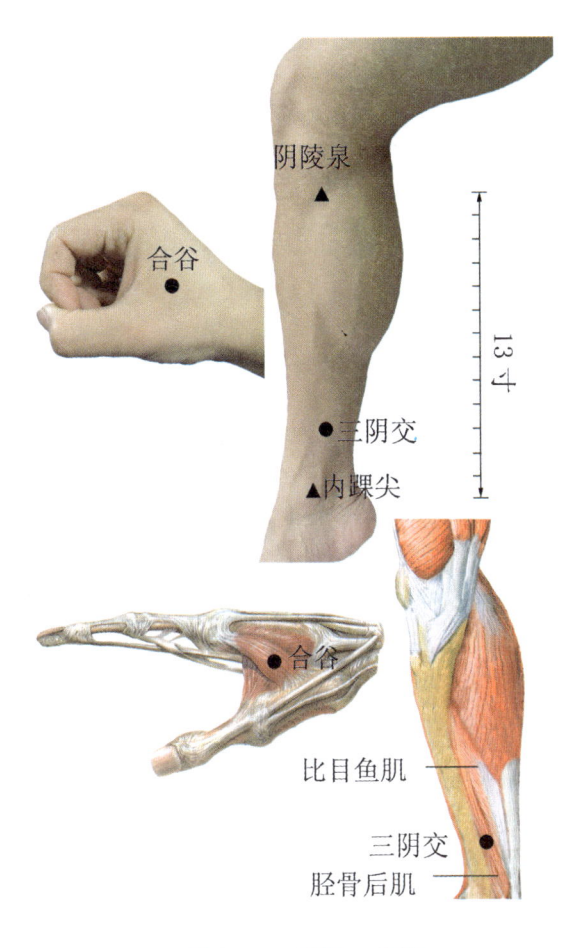

图 6－2　三阴交—合谷

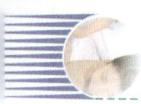

第三节　荨麻疹

组合穴　曲池—血海。
功　能　活血化瘀，疏风止痒。

曲池
【标准定位】在肘区，尺泽与肱骨外上髁上连线的中点处。
【毫针刺法】直刺 1.0～2.0 寸。

血海
【标准定位】屈膝，在大腿内侧，髌底内侧端上 2 寸，当股四头肌内侧头的隆起处。
【毫针刺法】直刺 1.0～2.0 寸，局部酸胀。

Section 3　Urticaria

Combination Point　Xuè Hǎi— Liáng Qiū.

Actions　Promoting blood flow and dispelling stasis, expelling wind and relieving itching.

LI 11 Qǔ Chí

Position　In the depression of the radial side of the transverse cubital crease when elbow flexed.

Acupuncture　Insert the needle perpendicularly 1.0～2.0 cun deep.

SP 10 Xuè Hǎi

Position　In the medial aspect of the thigh, 2 cun proximal to the medial edge of the patella, on the bulge of the medial portion of m. quadriceps femoris when the knee is flexed.

Acupuncture　Insert the needle perpendicularly 1.0～2.0 cun deep and stimulate until there is a sore and numbing sensation.

第六章 皮肤科疾病
Chapter 6　Dermatology diseases

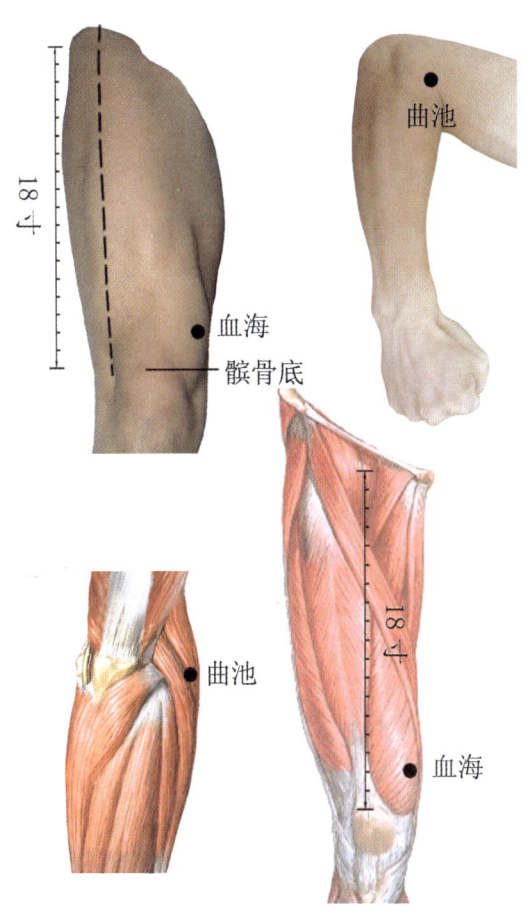

图6-3　曲池—血海

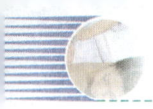

第四节 湿 疹

组合穴 曲池—阴陵泉。

功 能 健脾化湿,祛风止痒。

曲池

【标准定位】尺泽与肱骨外上髁上连线的中点处。

【毫针刺法】直刺1.0~2.0寸。

阴陵泉

【标准定位】在小腿内侧,胫骨内侧髁下缘与胫骨内侧缘之间的凹陷中。

【毫针刺法】直刺1.0~2.0寸。局部酸胀。

Section 4 Eczema

Combination Point Qǔ Chí—Yīn Líng Quán.

Actions Invigorating spleen and eliminating dampness, expelling wind and relieving itching.

LI 11 Qǔ Chí

Position In the depression of the radial side of the transverse cubital crease when elbow flexed.

Acupuncture Insert the needle perpendicularly 1.0~2.0 cun deep.

SP 9 Yīn Líng Quán

Position On the medial part of the lower leg, in the depression of the lower border of the medial condyle of the tibia.

Acupuncture Insert the needle perpendicularly 1.0~2.0 deep and stimulate until there is a sore and numbing sensation in the local area.

第六章 皮肤科疾病
Chapter 6 Dermatology diseases

阴陵泉

曲池

曲池

阴陵泉

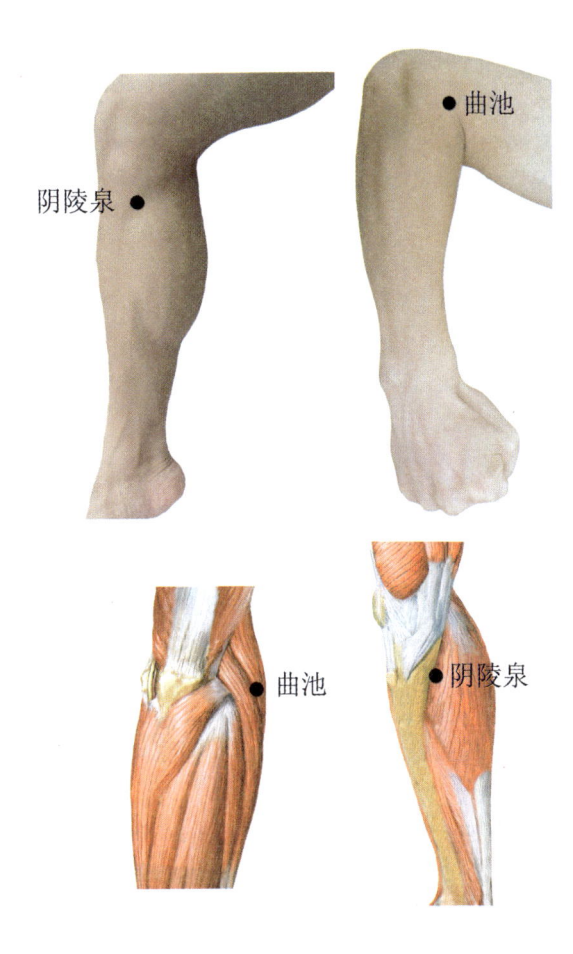

图 6-4 曲池（LI 11 Qǔ Chí）合谷（LI 4 Hé Gǔ）

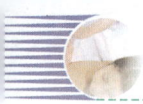

第五节 带状疱疹

组合穴 合谷—太冲。

功 能 清热泻火,解毒止痛。

合谷

【标准定位】在手背,第1、2掌骨间,第2掌骨桡侧的中点处。

【毫针刺法】直刺0.5~1.0寸。

太冲

【标准定位】在足背,当第1、2跖骨间,跖骨底结合部前方凹陷中。

【毫针刺法】向上斜刺0.5~1.0寸,局部酸胀。

Section 5　Zoster

Combination Point　Hé Gǔ—Tài Chōng.

Actions　Clearing heat and liver fire, alleviating pain.

LI 4 Hé Gǔ

Position　On the dorsum of the hand, between the first and second metacarpal bones, on the radial side of the middle of the second metacarpal bone.

Acupuncture　Insert the needle perpendicularly 0.5~1.0 cun deep.

LV 3 Tài Chōng

Position　On the dorsum of the foot, in the depression proximal to the first metatarsal space.

Acupuncture　Insert the needle obliquely upwards 0.5~1.0 cun deep and stimulate until there is a sore and numbing sensation.

第六章　皮肤科疾病
Chapter 6　Dermatology diseases

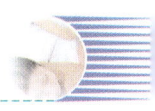

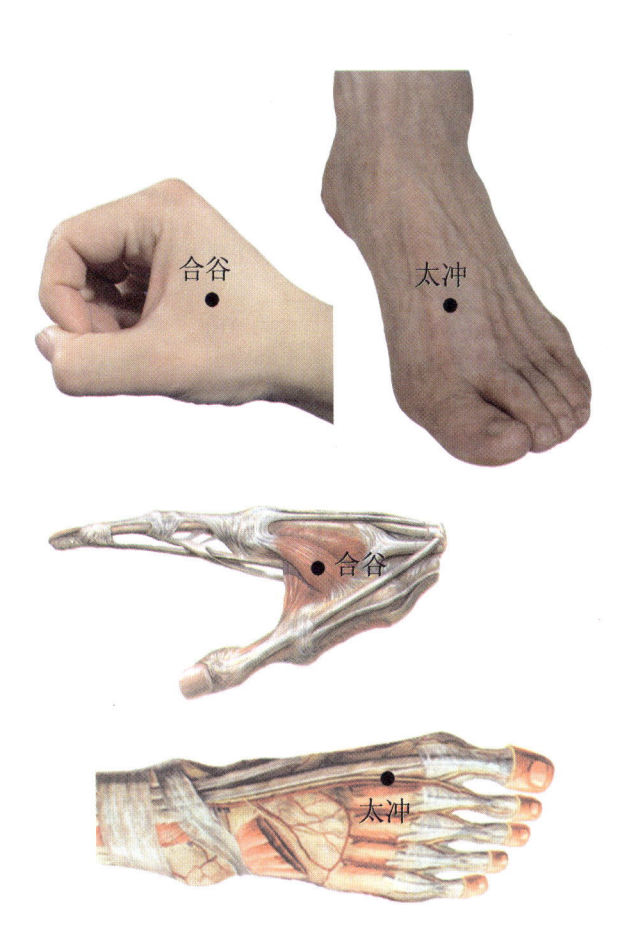

图 6-5　合谷—太冲

第六节　痤　疮

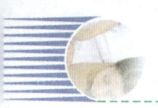

组合穴　风池—合谷。
功　能　疏风清热，行气活血。

风池
【标准定位】在颈后区，胸锁乳突肌上端与斜方肌上端之间的凹陷中。
【毫针刺法】向鼻尖方向斜刺 0.5~1.5 寸。

合谷
【标准定位】在手背，第 1、2 掌骨间，第 2 掌骨桡侧的中点处。
【毫针刺法】直刺 0.5~1.0 寸。

Section 6　Acne

Combination Point　Fēng Chí—Hé Gǔ.

Actions　Expelling wind and clearing heat, promoting qi and activating blood.

GB20 Fēng Chí

Position　On the nape, in the depression between m. sternocleidomastoideus and m. trapezius.

Acupuncture　Insert the needle obliquely toward the apex nasi 0.5~1.5 cun deep.

LI 4 Hé Gǔ

Position　On the dorsum of the hand, between the first and second metacarpal bones, on the radial side of the middle of the second metacarpal bone.

Acupuncture　Insert the needle perpendicularly 0.5~1.0 cun deep.

第六章 皮肤科疾病
Chapter 6　Dermatology diseases

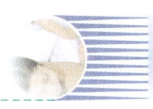

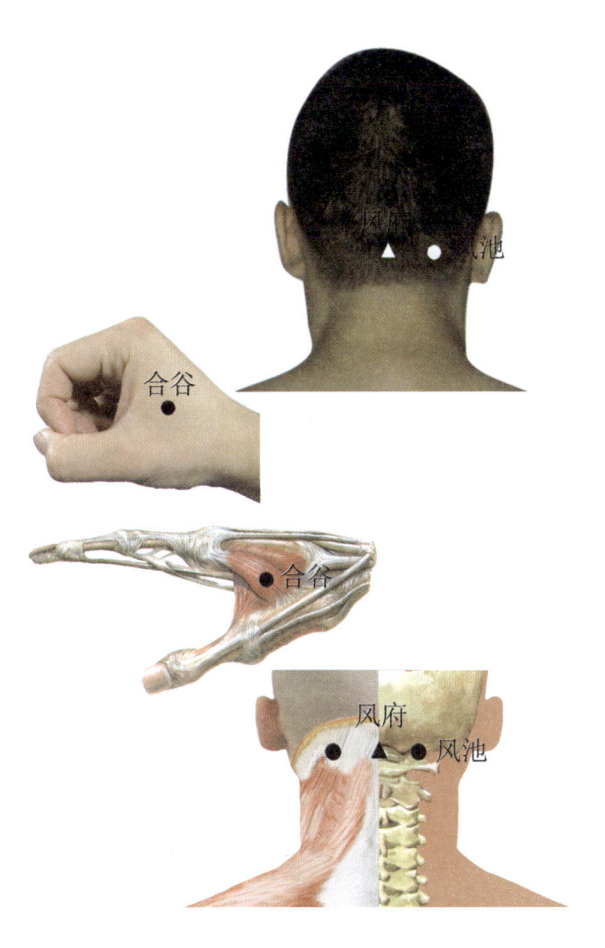

图 6-6　风池—合谷

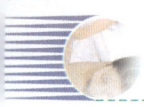

第七节 黄褐斑

组合穴 膈俞—肝俞。
功　能 疏肝理气，活血祛斑。

膈俞
【标准定位】在脊柱区，第7胸椎棘突下，后正中线旁开1.5寸。
【毫针刺法】向内斜刺0.5~0.8寸。

肝俞
【标准定位】第9胸椎棘突下，后正中线旁开1.5寸。
【毫针刺法】向内斜刺0.5~0.8寸。

Section 7　Chloasma

Combination Point　Gé Shū— Gān Shū.

Actions　Spreading liver and regulating qi.

BL 17 Gé Shū

Position　On the back, 1.5 cun lateral to the lower border of the spinous process of the seventh thoracic vertebra.

Acupuncture　Insert the needle obliquely towards the spine 0.5~0.8 cun deep.

BL 18 Gān Shū

Position　On the back, 1.5 cun lateral to the lower border of the spinous process of the ninth thoracic vertebra.

Acupuncture　Insert the needle obliquely towards the spine 0.5~0.8 cun deep.

第六章 皮肤科疾病
Chapter 6 Dermatology diseases

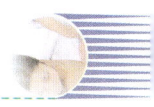

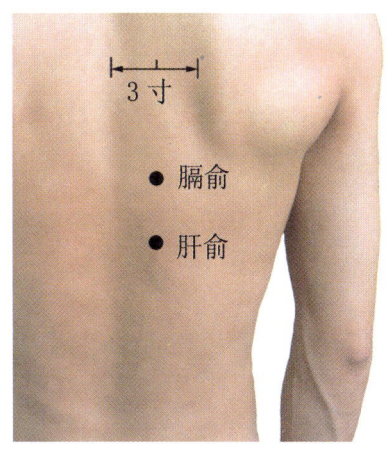

3寸

● 膈俞

● 肝俞

斜方肌

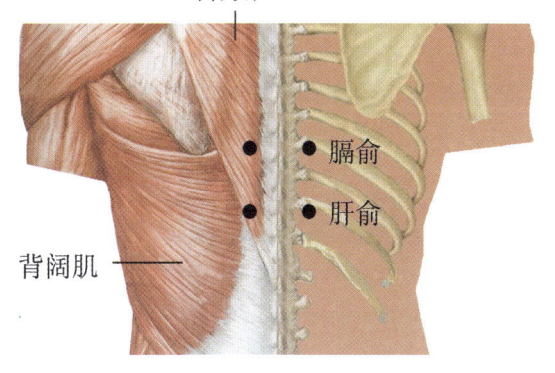

● 膈俞

● 肝俞

背阔肌

图 6-7 膈俞—肝俞

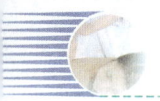

第七章　五官科病证
Chapter 7　ENT diseases

第一节　耳鸣、耳聋

组合穴　听宫—翳风。

功　能　通络聪耳。

听宫
【标准定位】下颌骨髁状突的后方，张口凹陷处。
【毫针刺法】张口位，直刺0.5~1.0寸。

翳风
【标准定位】耳垂后方，乳突下端前方凹陷中。
【毫针刺法】直刺0.8~1.2寸。

Section 1　Tinnitus, deafness

Combination Point　Tīng Gōng— Yì Fēng.

Actions　Activating the channel and benefiting the ears.

SI 19 Tīng Gōng

Position　On the face, anterior to the tragus, posterior to the condyloid process of lower jaw bone, in the depression when the mouth is opened.

Acupuncture　Insert the needle perpendicularly 0.5~1.0 cun deep.

SJ 17 Yì Fēng

Position　Posterior to the lobule of the ear, in the depression between the mastoid process and the angle of the mandible.

Acupuncture　Insert the needle perpendicularly 0.8~1.2 cun deep.

第七章 五官科病证
Chapter 7 ENT diseases

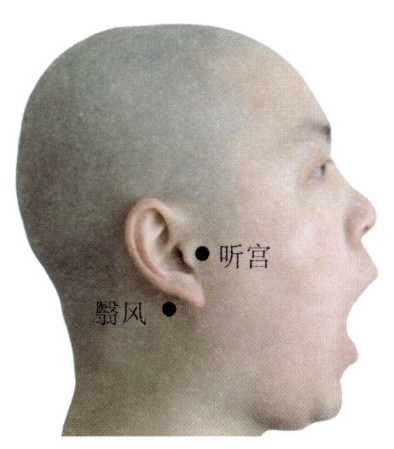

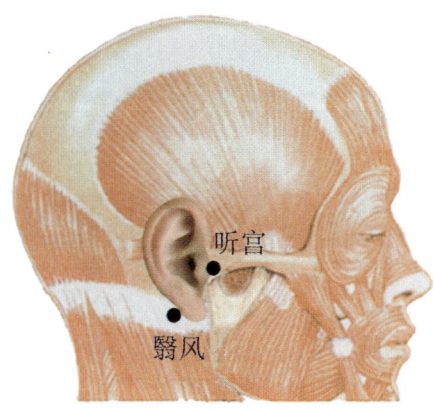

图7-1 听宫—翳风

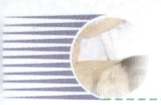

第二节 近 视

组合穴 睛明—风池。
功 能 通经活络,疏风明目。

睛明
【标准定位】目内眦内上方眶内侧壁凹陷中。
【毫针刺法】嘱患者闭目,医生用左手轻推眼球向外侧固定,右手持针缓慢刺入,紧靠眼眶直刺 0.3~0.8 寸,不提插,不捻转,局部酸胀。

风池
【标准定位】在颈后区,胸锁乳突肌上端与斜方肌上端之间的凹陷中。
【毫针刺法】向鼻尖方向斜刺 0.5~1.5 寸。

Section 2 Myopia

Combination Point Jīng Míng—Fēng Chí.

Actions Activiating the channel and collateral, expelling wind and improving vision.

BL 1 Jīng Míng

Position On the face, in the depression superior to the inner canthus.

Acupuncture Insert the needle slowly perpendicularly 0.3~0.8 cun deep while the eyes are closed by pushing the eyeball outwardly.

GB20 Fēng Chí

Position On the nape, in the depression between m. sternocleidomastoideus and m. trapezius.

Acupuncture Insert the needle obliquely toward the apex nasi 0.5~1.5 cun deep.

第七章　五官科病证
Chapter 7　ENT diseases

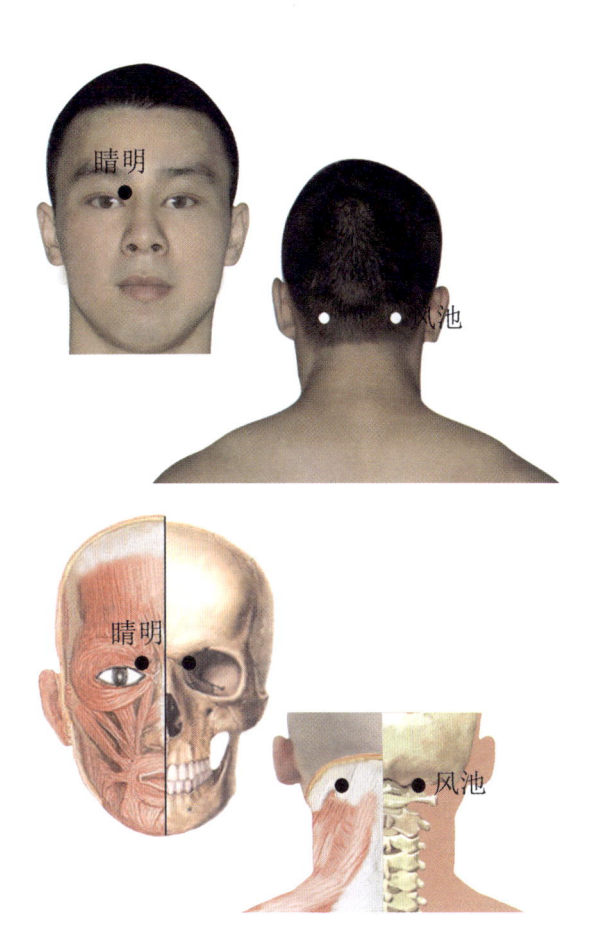

图 7-2　睛明—风池

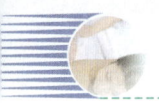

第三节 眼睑下垂

组合穴 攒竹—阳白。

功 能 舒筋通络,养筋提睑。

攒竹

【标准定位】在面部,当眉头陷中,眶上切迹处。

【毫针刺法】向外平刺0.3~0.5寸,局部酸胀。

阳白

【标准定位】在头部,瞳孔直上,眉上一寸。

【毫针刺法】向下平刺0.3~0.5寸,局部酸胀。

Section 3　Ptosis of eyelid

Combination Point　Cuán Zhú— Yáng Bái.

Actions　Relaxing sinews and activiating collaterals, nourishing the sinews to lift the eyelid.

BL 2 Cuán Zhú

Position　On the face, in the depression of the medial end of the eyebrow, in the supraorbital notch.

Acupuncture　Insert the needle subcutaneously 0.3~0.5 cun deep and stimulate until there is a sore and numbing sensation in the local area.

GB 14 Yáng Bái

Position　On the forehead, directly above the pupil, 1 cun superior to the eyebrow.

Acupuncture　Insert the needle subcutaneously 0.3~0.5 cun deep and stimulate until there is a sore and numbing sensation in the local area.

图7-3 攒竹—阳白

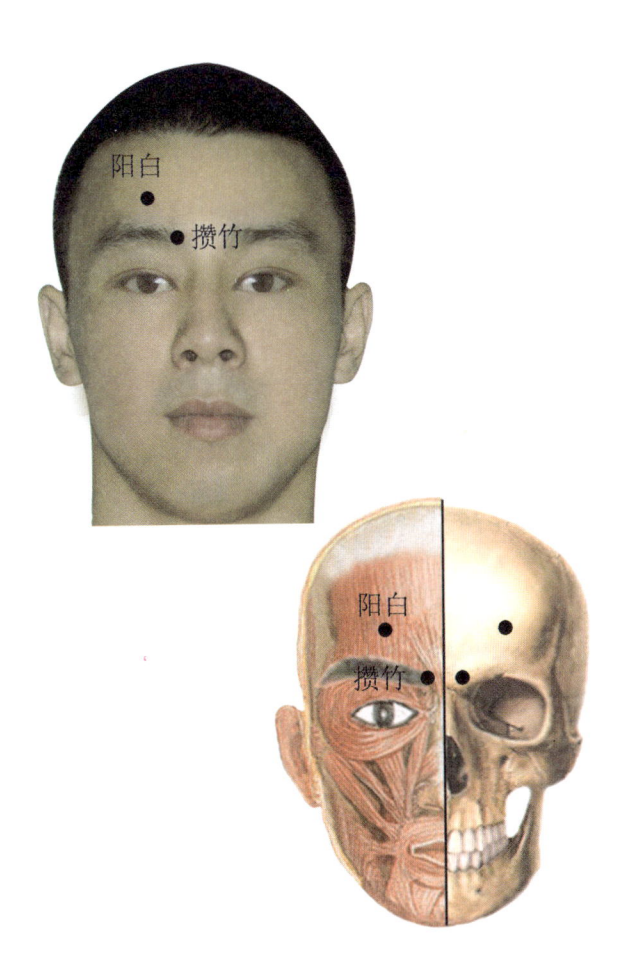

第四节　眼睑眲动

组合穴　合谷—太冲。
功　能　疏肝理气，熄风止痉。

合谷
【标准定位】在手背，第1、2掌骨间，第2掌骨桡侧的中点处。
【毫针刺法】直刺0.5~1.0寸。

太冲
【标准定位】在足背，当第1、2跖骨间，跖骨底结合部前方凹陷中。
【毫针刺法】向上斜刺0.5~1.0，局部酸胀。

Section 4　Eyelid run dynamic

Combination Point　Hé Gǔ—Tài Chōng.

Actions　Spreading Liver qi, calming liver wind and relieving convulsion.

LI 4 Hé Gǔ

Position　On the dorsum of the hand, between the first and second metacarpal bones, on the radial side of the middle of the second metacarpal bone.

Acupuncture　Insert the needle perpendicularly 0.5~1.0 cun deep.

LV 3 Tài Chōng

Position　On the dorsum of the foot, in the depression proximal to the first metatarsal space.

Acupuncture　Insert the needle obliquely upwards 0.5~1.0 cun deep and stimulate until there is a sore and numbing sensation.

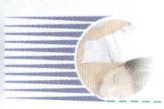

图 7-4 合谷—太冲

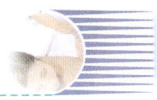

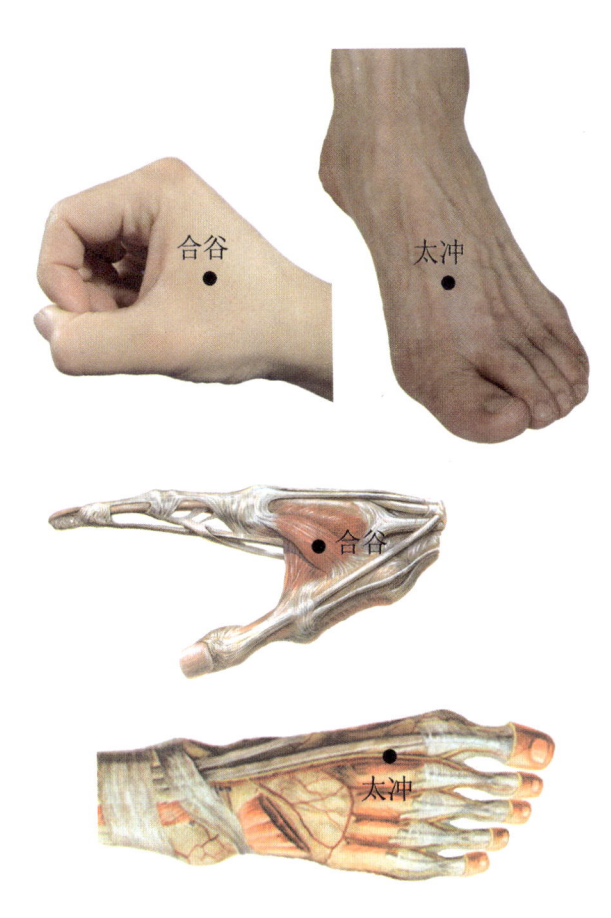

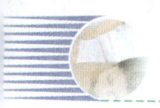

第五节 牙 痛

组合穴 下关—合谷。
功 能 舒筋活络止痛。

下关
【标准定位】当颧弓与下颌切迹所形成的凹陷处。
【毫针刺法】直刺0.8～1.2寸。

合谷
【标准定位】在手背,第1、2掌骨间,第2掌骨桡侧的中点处。
【毫针刺法】直刺0.5～1.0寸。

Section 5 Toothache

Combination Point Dì Cāng— Jiá Chē.

Actions Relaxing sinews, activiating collaterals, and alleviating pain.

ST 7 Xià Guān

Position In the depression between the zygomatic arch and mandibular notch in front of the ear.

Acupuncture Insert the needle perpendicularly 0.8～1.2 cun deep.

LI 4 Hé Gǔ

Position On the dorsum of the hand, between the first and second metacarpal bones, on the radial side of the middle of the second metacarpal bone.

Acupuncture Insert the needle perpendicularly 0.5～1.0 cun deep.

第七章　五官科病证
Chapter 7　ENT diseases

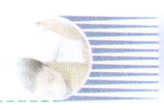

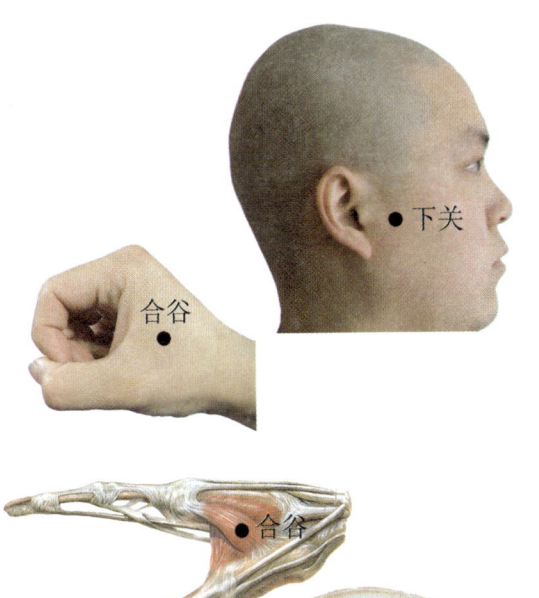

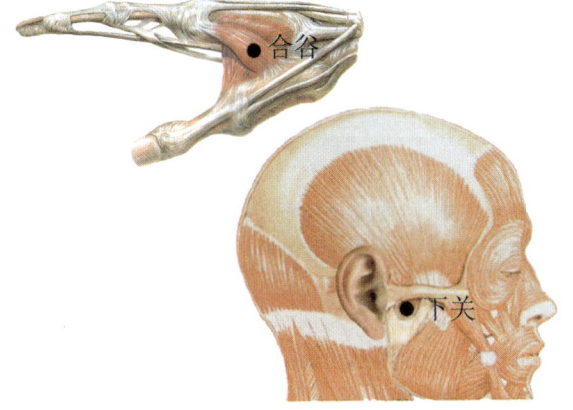

图 7-5　下关—合谷

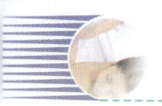

第六节　咽喉肿痛

组合穴　合谷—少商。

功　能　疏风清热，利咽止痛。

合谷

【标准定位】在手背，第1、2掌骨间，第2掌骨桡侧的中点处。

【毫针刺法】直刺0.5~1.0寸。

少商

【标准定位】在手指，拇指末节桡侧，指甲根角侧上方0.1寸（指寸）。

【毫针刺法】点刺出血。

Section 6　Sore throat

Combination Point　Hé Gǔ—Shào Shāng.

Actions　Expelling wind and clearing heat, relieving sore-throat.

LI 4 Hé Gǔ

Position　On the dorsum of the hand, between the first and second metacarpal bones, on the radial side of the middle of the second metacarpal bone.

Acupuncture　Insert the needle perpendicularly 0.5~1.0 cun deep.

LU 11 Shào Shāng

Position　On the radial side of the thumb, 0.1 cun lateral to the corner of the nail.

Acupuncture　Prick with three-edged needle and press tightly to expel drops of blood.

第七章　五官科病证
Chapter 7　ENT diseases

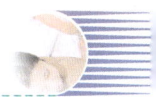

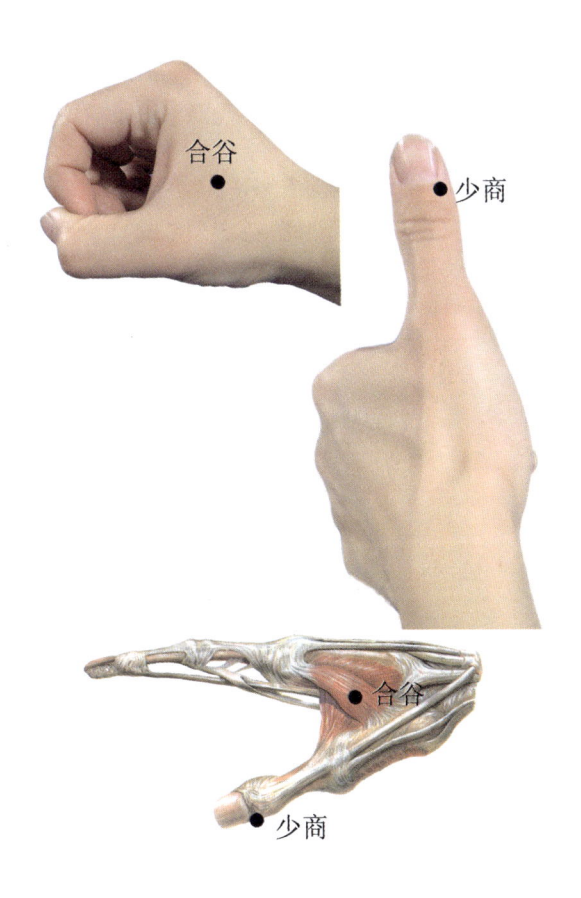

图 7-6　合谷—少商